CLINICAL DECISION MAKING

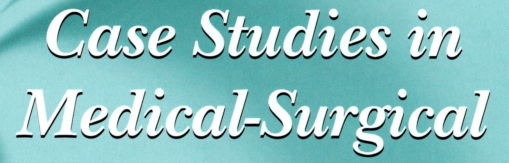

Case Studies in Medical-Surgical Nursing

SECOND EDITION

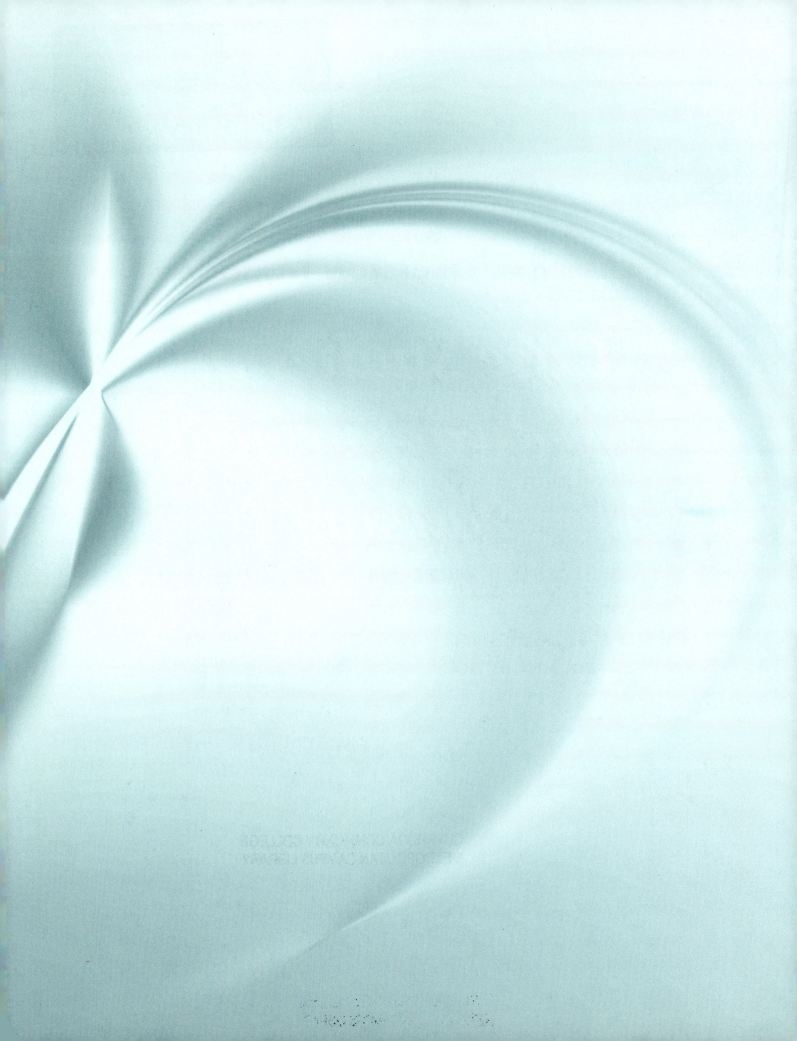

CLINICAL DECISION MAKING

Case Studies in Medical-Surgical Nursing

SECOND EDITION

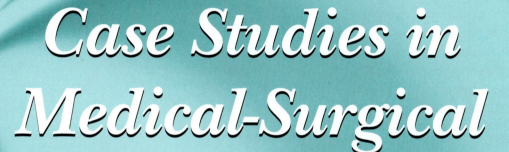

Gina M. Ankner

RN, MSN, ANP-BC

Revisions and New Cases Contributed by

Patricia M. Ahlschlager

RN, BSN, MSEd

and

Tammy J. Hale

RN, BSN

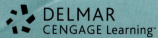

DELMAR
CENGAGE Learning™

Australia • Brazil • Japan • Korea • Mexico • Singapore • Spain • United Kingdom • United States

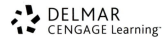
DELMAR
CENGAGE Learning™

Clinical Decision Making: Case Studies in Medical-Surgical Nursing, Second Edition
Gina M. Ankner, RN, MSN, ANP-BC

Vice President, Career Education and Training Solutions: Dave Garza

Director of Learning Solutions: Matthew Kane

Executive Editor: Steven Helba

Managing Editor: Marah Bellegarde

Senior Product Manager: Juliet Steiner

Editorial Assistant: Jennifer M. Wheaton

Vice President, Career Education and Training Solutions: Jennifer Baker

Marketing Director: Wendy Mapstone

Senior Marketing Manager: Michele McTighe

Marketing Coordinator: Scott Chrysler

Production Director: Carolyn Miller

Production Manager: Andrew Crouth

Content Project Management: PreMediaGlobal

Senior Art Director: Jack Pendleton

Technology Project Manager: Mary Colleen Liburdi

For product information and technology assistance, contact us at
Cengage Learning Customer & Sales Support, 1-800-354-9706

For permission to use material from this text or product, submit all requests online at **cengage.com/permissions**
Further permissions questions can be e-mailed to
permissionrequest@cengage.com

Library of Congress Control Number: 2010943448

ISBN-13: 978-1-111-13857-8

ISBN-10: 1-111-13857-5

Delmar
5 Maxwell Drive
Clifton Park, NY 12065-2919
USA

Cengage Learning is a leading provider of customized learning solutions with office locations around the globe, including Singapore, the United Kingdom, Australia, Mexico, Brazil, and Japan. Locate your local office at: **international.cengage.com/region**

Cengage Learning products are represented in Canada by Nelson Education, Ltd.

To learn more about Delmar, visit **www.cengage.com/delmar**

Purchase any of our products at your local college store or at our preferred online store **www.cengagebrain.com**

Notice to the Reader

Publisher does not warrant or guarantee any of the products described herein or perform any independent analysis in connection with any of the product information contained herein. Publisher does not assume, and expressly disclaims, any obligation to obtain and include information other than that provided to it by the manufacturer. The reader is expressly warned to consider and adopt all safety precautions that might be indicated by the activities described herein and to avoid all potential hazards. By following the instructions contained herein, the reader willingly assumes all risks in connection with such instructions. The publisher makes no representations or warranties of any kind, including but not limited to, the warranties of fitness for particular purpose or merchantability, nor are any such representations implied with respect to the material set forth herein, and the publisher takes no responsibility with respect to such material. The publisher shall not be liable for any special, consequential, or exemplary damages resulting, in whole or part, from the readers' use of, or reliance upon, this material.

Printed in the United States of America
1 2 3 4 5 6 7 15 14 13 12 11

Contents

Reviewers

Dee Adkins, MSN, RN
Harrison College
Indianapolis Indiana

Patricia N. Allen, MSN, APRN-BC
Clinical Assistant Professor
Indiana University School of Nursing
Bloomington, Indiana

Bonita E. Broyles, RN, BSN, PhD
Associate Degree Nursing Faculty
Piedmont Community College
Roxboro, North Carolina

Joyce Campbell, MSN, APRN, BC, CCRN
Associate Professor
Chattanooga State Community College
Chattanooga, Tennessee

Fran Cherkis, MS, RN, CNE
Farmingdale State College
Farmingdale, New York

Marianne Curia, MSN, RN
Assistant Professor
University of St. Francis
Joliet, Illinois

Karen K. Gerbasich, RN, MSN
Faculty Assistant Professor
Ivy Tech Community College
South Bend, Indiana

Amanda M. Reynolds, MSN
Associate Professor
Grambling State University
Grambling, Louisiana

Preface

Delmar's Case Study Series was created to encourage nurses to bridge the gap between content knowledge and clinical application. The products within the series represent the most innovative and comprehensive approach to nursing case studies ever developed. Each title has been authored by experienced nurse educators and clinicians who understand the complexity of nursing practice, as well as the challenges of teaching and learning. All the cases are based on real-life clinical scenarios and demand thought and "action" from the nurse. Each case brings the user into the clinical setting and invites the user to employ the nursing process while considering all the variables that influence the client's condition and the care to be provided. Each case also represents a unique set of variables, to offer a breadth of learning experiences and to capture the reality of nursing practice. In order to gauge the progression of a user's knowledge and critical thinking ability, the cases have been categorized by difficulty level. Every section begins with basic cases and proceeds to more advanced scenarios, thereby presenting opportunities for learning and practice for both students and professionals.

All the cases have been reviewed by experts to ensure that as many variables as possible are represented in a truly realistic manner and that each case reflects consistency with realities of modern nursing practice.

Praise for Delmar's Case Study Series

"[This text's] strength is the large variety of case studies—it seemed to be all inclusive. Another strength is the extensiveness built into each case study. You can almost see this person as they enter the ED because of the descriptions that are given."

—MARY BETH KIEFNER, RN, MS,
Nursing Program Director/Nursing Faculty,
Illinois Central College

"The cases . . . reflect the complexity of nursing practice. They are an excellent way to refine critical-thinking skills."

—DARLA R. URA, MA, RN, APRN, BC,
Clinical Associate Professor, Adult and Elder
Health Department, School of Nursing,
Emory University

"The case studies are very comprehensive and allow the undergraduate student an opportunity to apply knowledge gained in the classroom to a potentially real clinical situation."

—TAMELLA LIVENGOOD, APRN, BC, MSN, FNP,
Nursing Faculty, Northwestern Michigan College

"These cases and how you have approached them definitely stimulate the students to use critical-thinking skills. I thought the questions asked really pushed the students to think deeply and thoroughly."

—JOANNE SOLCHANY, PhD, ARNP, RN, CS,
Assistant Professor, Family & Child Nursing,
University of Washington, Seattle

"The use of case studies is pedagogically sound and very appealing to students and instructors. I think that some instructors avoid them because of the challenge of case development. You have provided the material for them."

—NANCY L. OLDENBURG, RN, MS, CPNP,
Clinical Instructor, Northern Illinois University

"[The author] has done an excellent job of assisting students to engage in critical thinking. I am very impressed with the cases, questions, and content. I rarely ask that students buy more than one . . . book . . . but, in this instance, I can't wait until this book is published."

—DEBORAH J. PERSELL, MSN, RN, CPNP,
Assistant Professor, Arkansas State University

"This is a groundbreaking book. . . . This book should be a required text for all undergraduate and graduate nursing programs and should be well-received by faculty."

—JANE H. BARNSTEINER, PhD, RN, FAAN,
Professor of Pediatric Nursing, University of
Pennsylvania School of Nursing

How to Use This Book

Every case begins with a table of variables that is encountered in practice, and that must be understood by the nurse in order to provide appropriate care to the client. Categories of variables include gender, age, setting, ethnicity, cultural considerations, preexisting conditions, coexisting conditions, communication considerations, disability considerations, socioeconomic considerations, spiritual/religious considerations, pharmacologic considerations, legal considerations, ethical considerations, alternative therapy, prioritization considerations, and delegation considerations. If a case involves a variable that is considered to have a significant impact on care, the specific variable is included in the table. This allows the user an "at a glance" view of the issues that will need to be considered to provide care to the client in the scenario. The table of variables is followed by a presentation of the case, including the history of the client, current condition, clinical setting, and professionals involved. A series of questions follows each case that require the user to consider how she or he would handle the issues presented within the scenario. Suggested answers and rationales are provided in the accompanying *Instructor's Manual* for remediation and discussion.

Organization

Cases are grouped according to body system and are reorganized in this edition for a head-to-toe approach. Within each part, cases are organized by difficulty level from easy, to moderate, to difficult. This classification is somewhat subjective, but it is based upon a developed standard. In general, the difficulty level has been determined by the number of variables that affect the case and the complexity of the client's condition. Colored tabs are used to allow the user to distinguish the difficulty levels more easily. A comprehensive table of variables is also provided for reference to allow the user to quickly select cases containing a particular variable of care.

While every effort has been made to group cases into the most applicable body system, the scope of many of the cases may include more than one body system. In such instances, the case will still only appear in the section for one of the body systems addressed. The cases are fictitious; however, they are based on actual problems and/or situations the nurse will encounter.

Features

- Reflecting real-world practice, the cases are designed to help the user sharpen critical thinking skills and gain hands-on experience applying what the user has learned.

- Providing comprehensive coverage, 43 detailed case studies cover a wide range of topics.

- Case studies progress by difficulty level, from easy to moderate to difficult, which can be identified by colored tabs.

- Written by nurses with modern clinical experience, these cutting-edge cases are relevant to the real-world challenges and pressures of practice—offering insight into the realities of today's profession.

- Cases include a wide assortment of variables related to client diversity, prioritization, and legal and ethical considerations.

New to This Edition

- Cases are completely updated, reflecting the latest practices in the field.

- Four new case studies cover Bell's Palsy, Glaucoma, Renal Calculi, and Septic Shock.

- Body systems have been reorganized to follow a head-to-toe approach.

- Nursing diagnoses are updated to reflect NANDA International's *Nursing Diagnoses: Definitions and Classifications 2009–2011*.

Also Available

Instructor's Manual to Accompany Clinical Decision Making: Case Studies in Medical-Surgical Nursing, Second Edition, by Gina M. Ankner

ISBN-10: 1-111-13858-3

ISBN-13: 978-1-111-13858-5

This instructor's manual provides suggested answers and rationales, with references, to each of the case studies in this book. Instructors can use this to evaluate and assess student responses to cases, or as a discussion tool in the classroom.

Clinical Decision Making: Online Case Studies in Medical-Surgical Nursing, Second Edition

A convenient way for you to use these popular case studies online, please visit www.cengagebrain.com for more information on this resource.

Delmar's Case Study Series: Medical-Surgical Nursing, Second Edition, by Gina M. Ankner

ISBN-10: 1-111-13859-1

ISBN-13: 978-1-111-13859-2

Following the same general case study model, this resource provides an additional 22 case studies based on real-life clinical scenarios that demand critical thinking from the nurse. Suggested answers and rationales are provided immediately following each case to support remediation, review, and discussion.

Acknowledgments

Special thanks go to Patricia M. Ahlschlager and Tammy J. Hale for their hard work revising and updating these cases and contributing the new case studies. Thank you to the publishing team at Delmar Cengage Learning: Steven Helba,

Juliet Steiner, Jennifer Wheaton, Jack Pendleton, and Jim Zayicek. Many thanks to those individuals who willingly shared their personal stories so that future nurses could learn from them. The input from students, friends, and family was invaluable, especially the generosity of Kimberly Dodd, MD, and Kathleen Elliott, ANP, BC, whose contributions and support exemplify friendship and professional collaboration. With great appreciation, I wish to acknowledge the reviewers for the constructive comments and suggestions that helped to enhance the educational value of each case.

About the Author

Gina Ankner, RN, MSN, ANP-BC, is senior nurse coordinator and program director for the Specialty Care in Pregnancy Program (SCIPP) in the Department of Medicine at Women & Infants Hospital of Rhode Island. The only program of its kind in the United States, SCIPP brings a multidisciplinary team together to consult on cases of women whose pregnancy, or plan for pregnancy, is complicated by a medical condition. She is also responsible for outreach and new program development for the Department of Medicine. Prior to her current position at Women & Infants Hospital, she taught medical-surgical nursing for ten years at the University of Massachusetts Dartmouth College of Nursing. Ankner earned her bachelor's and master's degrees in nursing from Boston College.

Note from the Author

My students were the inspiration for this book. With rare exception, each case study is based on a client that a student cared for. Through the student's eyes, I share stories of men and women who have turned to their nurses for care and support during their illness. Perhaps when reading a scenario, you will think, "It would not happen like that." Please know that it did and that it will. The most enjoyable part of writing each case was the realization that another nursing student will learn from the experience of a peer. The intent was not only to provide the more common patient scenarios, but also to present actual cases that encourage critical thinking and prompt a student to ask "what if?"

The wonderful thing about a case study is that possibilities for learning abound! These cases provide a foundation upon which endless knowledge can be built. So be creative—change a client's gender, age, or ethnicity, pose new questions, but, most importantly, enjoy the journey of becoming a better nurse.

The author welcomes comments via e-mail at MedSurgCases@yahoo.com.

Comprehensive Table of Variables

CASE STUDY	GENDER	AGE	SETTING	ETHNICITY	CULTURE	PREEXISTING CONDITIONS	COEXISTING CONDITIONS	COMMUNICATION	DISABILITY	SOCIOECONOMIC STATUS	SPIRITUALITY	PHARMACOLOGIC	LEGAL	ETHICAL	ALTERNATIVE THERAPY	PRIORITIZATION	DELEGATION
Part One: The Cardiovascular System & the Blood																	
1	F	20	Hospital	Asian American						X		X	X			X	
2	M	58	Rehabilitation unit	Asian American		X				X		X				X	
3	F	71	Hospital	Russian		X	X			X		X			X		
4	F	88	Primary care	White American	X	X						X				X	
5	M	42	Hospital	White American		X	X		X	X			X	X			
6	F	67	Hospital	Black American	X	X						X				X	
7	F	70	Home	Black American	X	X				X		X					
8	F	20	Hospital	Black American	X	X				X		X			X		
9	F	55	Hospital	White American		X	X					X	X				
Part Two: The Respiratory System																	
1	F	38	Walk-in	White American		X				X		X				X	
2	M	25	Hospital	Black American								X				X	
3	M	75	Hospital	Jewish American	X	X	X		X		X	X			X	X	
4	M	67	Primary care	White American		X				X							
Part Three: The Nervous/Neurological System																	
1	F	43	Emergency department	White American		X				X		X			X		
2	F	59	Hospital	Black American		X				X		X			X		
3	M	85	Long-term care	Native American	X	X	X	X	X	X							
4	F	92	Hospital	White American		X	X					X	X				
5	F	35	Hospital	White American	X	X				X		X				X	
6	M	73	Home	White American				X	X	X		X	X		X	X	X
Part Four: The Sensory System																	
1	M	73	Outpatient clinic	Black American		X	X			X	X	X					
Part Five: The Integumentary System																	
1	F	70	Home	White American		X	X			X	X					X	
2	M	57	Hospital	White American		X						X			X	X	X
3	F	72	Hospital	White American		X			X	X		X	X	X		X	X
4	M	32	Primary care	White American						X		X					
5	M	55	Hospital	Black American		X	X		X			X				X	

CASE STUDY	GENDER	AGE	SETTING	ETHNICITY	CULTURE	PREEXISTING CONDITIONS	COEXISTING CONDITIONS	COMMUNICATION	DISABILITY	SOCIOECONOMIC STATUS	SPIRITUALITY	PHARMACOLOGIC	LEGAL	ETHICAL	ALTERNATIVE THERAPY	PRIORITIZATION	DELEGATION
Part Six: The Digestive System																	
1	F	46	Hospital	White American			X			X		X					
2	F	46	Hospital	White American			X			X	X	X	X			X	X
3	F	33	Hospital	White American			X			X	X	X					X
4	M	44	Hospital	White American		X	X					X				X	
5	F	63	Hospital	White American		X	X		X	X		X					X
Part Seven: The Urinary System																	
1	F	35	Hospital	Native American	X			X		X		X				X	
2	F	56	Hospital	Hispanic		X	X			X		X				X	
3	F	56	Hospital	Hispanic		X	X			X				X		X	X
Part Eight: The Endocrine/Metabolic System																	
1	M	91	Long-term care	White American			X		X	X		X					X
2	M	61	Hospital	Mexican American	X	X	X	X		X		X	X	X	X		X
3	F	88	Hospital	White American			X					X					
Part Nine: The Skeletal System																	
1	M	81	Hospital	Portuguese	X	X	X	X	X	X			X	X			
2	F	77	Hospital	Black American	X	X	X			X	X	X					X
3	M	73	Hospital	White American			X					X					
Part Ten: The Muscular System																	
1	M	81	Hospital	White American		X	X			X	X	X	X				X
2	F	48	Primary care	White American			X		X	X		X			X		
Part Eleven: The Reproductive System																	
1	F	45	Hospital	Black American			X			X		X				X	X
Part Twelve: Multi-System Failure																	
1	F	74	Intensive care unit	White American		X				X		X					

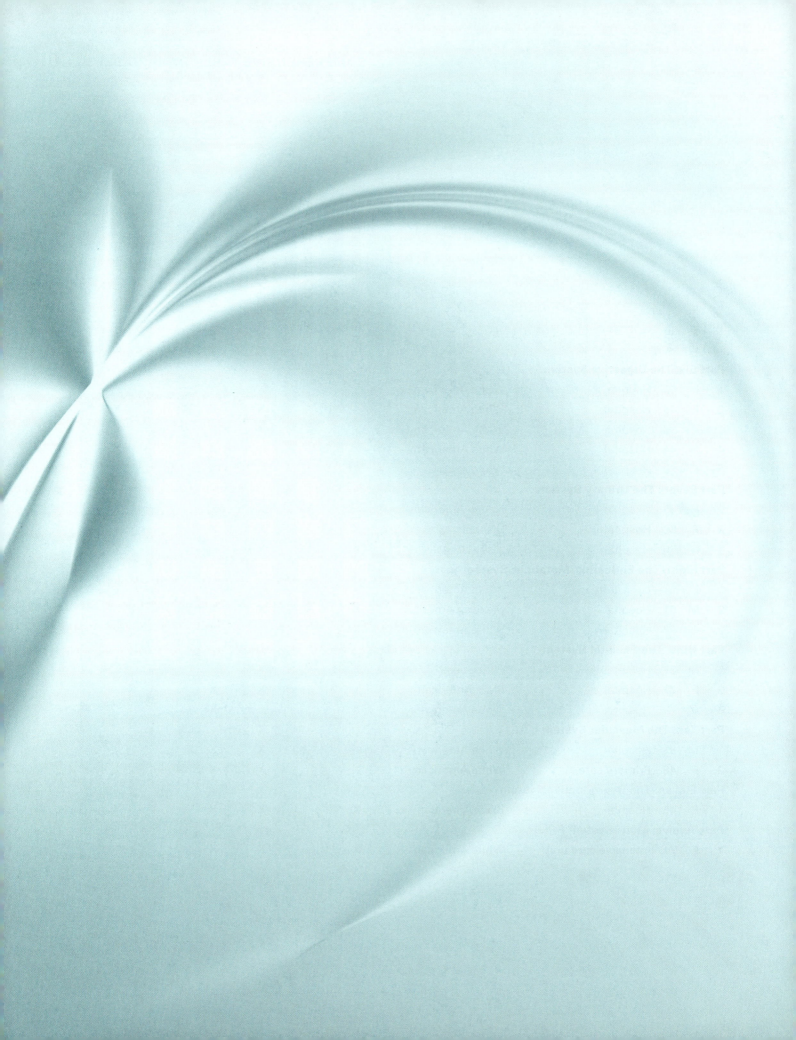

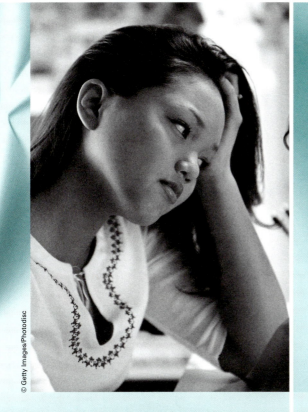

The Cardiovascular System & the Blood

EASY

GENDER	**SPIRITUAL/RELIGIOUS**
Female	
AGE	**PHARMACOLOGIC**
20	■ Zidovudine (Retrovir); lamivudine (Epivir); didanosine (Videx); indinavir sulfate (Crixivan)
SETTING	**LEGAL**
■ Hospital	■ Blood-borne pathogen exposure; incident (occurrence or variance) report
ETHNICITY	
■ Asian American	**ETHICAL**
CULTURAL CONSIDERATIONS	**ALTERNATIVE THERAPY**
PREEXISTING CONDITION	**PRIORITIZATION**
COEXISTING CONDITION	■ Immediate assessment of injury is necessary
COMMUNICATION	**DELEGATION**
DISABILITY	
SOCIOECONOMIC	
■ Cost of needle stick injury testing, treatment, and follow-up	

THE CARDIOVASCULAR SYSTEM & THE BLOOD

Level of difficulty: Easy

Overview: This case requires that the student nurse recognize the appropriate interventions following a needle stick injury. Her risk of blood-borne pathogen exposure is considered. Testing, treatment, suggested follow-up, and the cost associated are discussed. An incident (occurrence or variance) report is completed.

Client Profile

Bethany is a 20-year-old nursing student. Although she has practiced the intramuscular injection technique in the nursing laboratory, she is nervous about giving her first intramuscular injection to a "real" client.

Case Study

Bethany has reviewed the procedure and the selected intramuscular site landmark technique. She follows all the proper steps, including donning gloves. The syringe was equipped with a safety device to cover the needle after injection, but after giving the injection, before the instructor can stop her, Bethany attempts to recap the needle and sticks herself with the needle through her glove. She is embarrassed to say anything in front of the client so she removes her gloves and washes her hands. Once outside the client's room, Bethany shows the nursing instructor her finger. There is blood visible on her finger where she stuck herself.

Questions

1. What should Bethany do first?

2. Discuss the appropriate interventions that the clinical agency should initiate following Bethany's needle stick injury.

3. What is the recommended drug therapy based on the level of risk of HIV exposure?

4. Which form(s) of hepatitis is Bethany most at risk for contracting? Discuss her level of risk of the form(s) of hepatitis you identified, as well as the risk of infection with HIV resulting from this needle stick.

5. Can the client's blood be tested for communicable diseases if the client does not give consent?

6. What will be the recommendations for Bethany's follow-up antibody testing?

7. HIV test results are reported as *positive, negative,* or *indeterminate*. What does each result mean?

8. What is an incident (occurrence or variance) report, and why should Bethany and her nursing instructor complete one?

9. Discuss how Bethany could have prevented this needle stick injury.

10. Bethany's nursing instructor decides to share information with the nursing students about OSHA's Needlestick Safety and Prevention Act. Explain OSHA's role and the safety and prevention act.

11. Discuss who is most likely responsible for the expense of Bethany's care immediately following the needle stick and any follow-up care. What risks are presented if the expense is prohibitive?

12. Identify three potential nursing diagnoses appropriate for Bethany.

Mr. Luke

GENDER

Male

AGE

58

SETTING

- Outpatient rehabilitation unit

ETHNICITY

- Asian American

CULTURAL CONSIDERATIONS

PREEXISTING CONDITION

- Left total knee replacement (TKR) five days ago

COEXISTING CONDITION

COMMUNICATION

DISABILITY

SOCIOECONOMIC

- Smokes one pack of cigarettes per day

SPIRITUAL/RELIGIOUS

PHARMACOLOGIC

- Enoxaparin (Lovenox); dalteparin sodium (Fragmin); warfarin sodium (Coumadin); nicotine transdermal system (Nicoderm CQ); acetylsalicylic acid (aspirin, ASA); dextran (Macrodex, Gentran)

LEGAL

ETHICAL

ALTERNATIVE THERAPY

PRIORITIZATION

- Prevention of pulmonary embolism (PE)

DELEGATION

THE CARDIOVASCULAR SYSTEM & THE BLOOD

Level of difficulty: Easy

Overview: This case requires the nurse to recognize the symptoms of a deep vein thrombosis (DVT), understand the diagnostic tests used to confirm this diagnosis, and discuss the rationale for a treatment plan. Nursing diagnoses to include in the client's plan of care are prioritized.

Client Profile

Mr. Luke is a 58-year-old man who is currently a client on an outpatient rehabilitation unit following a left total knee replacement (TKR) five days ago. This afternoon during physical therapy he complained that his left leg was unusually painful when walking. His left leg was noted to have increased swelling from the prior day. He was sent to the emergency department to be examined.

Case Study

Mr. Luke's vital signs are temperature 98.1°F (36.7°C), blood pressure 110/50, pulse 65, and respiratory rate of 19. His oxygen saturation is 98% on room air. The result of a serum D-dimer is 7 µg/mL. Physical exam reveals that his left calf circumference measurement is ¾ of an inch larger than his right leg calf circumference. Mr. Luke's left calf is warmer to the touch than his right. He will have a noninvasive compression/doppler flow study (doppler ultrasound) to rule out a DVT in his left leg.

Questions

1. The health care provider in the emergency department chooses not to assess Mr. Luke for a positive Homan's sign. What is a Homan's sign and why did the health care provider defer this assessment?

2. Discuss the diagnostic cues gathered during Mr. Luke's examination in the emergency department that indicate a possible DVT.

3. Discuss Virchow's triad and the physiological development of a DVT.

4. The nurse who cared for Mr. Luke immediately following his knee surgery, when writing the postoperative plan of care, included appropriate interventions to help prevent venous thromboembolism. Discuss five nonpharmacological interventions the nurse included in the plan.

5. Discuss the common pharmacologic therapy options for postsurgical clients to help reduce the risk of a DVT.

6. Mr. Luke's noninvasive compression/doppler flow study (doppler ultrasound) shows a small thrombus located below the popliteal vein of his left leg. While a positive DVT is always of concern, why is the health care provider relieved that the thrombus is located there and not in the popliteal vein?

7. Mr. Luke was admitted to the hospital for observation overnight. He is being discharged back to the rehabilitation unit with the following prescribed discharge instructions:

(a) bed rest with bathroom privileges (BRP) with elevation of left leg for 72 hours;

(b) thromboembolic devices (TEDs);

(c) continue with enoxaparin 75 mg subcutaneously (SQ) every 12 hours;

(d) warfarin sodium 5 mg by mouth (PO) per day starting tomorrow;

(e) nicotine transdermal system 21 mg per day for 6 weeks, then 14 mg per day for 2 weeks, and then 7 mg per day for 2 weeks;

(f) acetylsalicylic acid 325 mg PO once daily;

(g) prothrombin time (PT) and international normalized ratio (INR) daily;

(h) occult blood (OB) test of stools;

(i) have vitamin K available; and

(j) vital signs every four hours.

Provide a rationale for each of the prescribed discharge instructions.

9. Prioritize five nursing diagnoses to include in Mr. Luke's plan of care when he returns to the rehabilitation unit.

10. What is an inferior vena cava (IVC) filter and for which clients is this filter indicated?

11. Discuss the symptoms the nurse at the rehabilitation center should watch for that could indicate that Mr. Luke has developed a pulmonary embolism (PE).

12. Because of the DVT, Mr. Luke is at risk for postphlebitic syndrome (also called post-thrombotic syndrome or PTS). Discuss the incidence, cause, symptoms, and prevention of this potential long-term complication.

GENDER

Female

AGE

71

SETTING

- Hospital

ETHNICITY

- Russian

CULTURAL CONSIDERATIONS

PREEXISTING CONDITIONS

- Heart failure (HF, CHF); pneumonia; chronic obstructive pulmonary disease (COPD); gastroesophageal reflux disease (GERD)

COEXISTING CONDITION

COMMUNICATION

- Russian speaking only; daughter speaks English

DISABILITY

SOCIOECONOMIC

- Lives with daughter's family

SPIRITUAL/RELIGIOUS

PHARMACOLOGIC

- Digoxin (Lanoxin); potassium chloride (KCl); atropine sulfate (Atropine); digoxin immune fab (Digibind)

LEGAL

ETHICAL

ALTERNATIVE THERAPY

- Licorice (glycyrrhiza, licorice root)

PRIORITIZATION

DELEGATION

THE CARDIOVASCULAR SYSTEM & THE BLOOD

Level of difficulty: Easy

Overview: This case requires that the nurse be knowledgeable regarding the action and pharmacokinetics of digoxin. The nurse must recognize the symptoms of digoxin toxicity and discuss appropriate treatment. The interaction between digoxin and an herbal remedy is considered. Priority nursing diagnoses for this client are identified.

Client Profile

Mrs. Kidway is a 71-year-old woman who lives at home with her daughter's family. Her daily medications prior to admission include digoxin 0.125 mg once a day.

Case Study

Mrs. Kidway arrives in the emergency room with her daughter who explains, "She was fine this morning but then this afternoon she developed terrible abdominal pain and got short of breath." Mrs. Kidway is lethargic. Her physical examination is unremarkable except for facial grimacing when palpating her abdomen. She is afebrile with a blood pressure of 105/50, pulse 60, and respiratory rate 18. Blood work on admission reveals a digoxin level of 3.8 ng/mL.

Questions

1. How does digoxin work in the body?

2. Why is Mrs. Kidway taking digoxin?

3. Given Mrs. Kidway's digoxin level, briefly explain what electrolyte imbalance is of concern.

4. During a nursing assessment of Mrs. Kidway's current medications, the nurse asks if Mrs. Kidway takes any over-the-counter medications or herbal remedies. Mrs. Kidway's daughter says, "Is licorice considered an herbal remedy? My mother started taking licorice capsules about a month ago because we heard that licorice helps decrease heartburn." Does licorice interact with digoxin? If so, explain.

5. Discuss what the terms *loading dose* and *steady state* indicate.

6. What are the onset, peak, and duration times of digoxin when it is taken orally?

7. If Mrs. Kidway was having difficulty swallowing her digoxin capsule and her health care provider changed her prescription to the elixir form of digoxin, theoretically would she still receive 0.125 mg?

8. What is a medication's "half-life"? What is the half-life of digoxin? Theoretically, if Mrs. Kidway took her digoxin at 8:00 A.M. on a Monday, when will 75% of the digoxin be cleared from her body according to the half-life? Since the half-life of digoxin is prolonged in the elderly, use the high end of the range of digoxin's half-life.

9. What is the normal therapeutic range of serum digoxin for a client taking this medication?

10. What symptoms may be noted when digoxin levels are at toxic levels?

11. At what serum digoxin range do cardiac dysrhythmias appear and what is the critical value for adults?

12. Mrs. Kidway's heart rate drops to 50 beats per minute. Her potassium is 2.1 mEq/L. She is given four vials of intravenous digoxin immune fab (reconstituted with sterile water) and admitted to the intensive care unit for monitoring. Discuss how her digoxin toxicity will be treated.

13. What are the two highest priority nursing diagnoses appropriate for Mrs. Kidway's plan of care?

Mrs. Andersson

GENDER

Female

AGE

88

SETTING

■ Primary care

ETHNICITY

■ White American

CULTURAL CONSIDERATIONS

■ Swedish; increased risk of pernicious anemia

PREEXISTING CONDITIONS

■ Small bowel obstruction (SBO) with subsequent bowel resection; diverticulitis

COEXISTING CONDITION

COMMUNICATION

DISABILITY

SOCIOECONOMIC

SPIRITUAL/RELIGIOUS

PHARMACOLOGIC

■ Cyanocobalamin (oral vitamin B_{12}); cyanocobalamin crystalline (injectable vitamin B_{12}); cyanocobalamin nasal gel (Nascobal); hydrochloric acid (HCl)

LEGAL

ETHICAL

ALTERNATIVE THERAPY

PRIORITIZATION

■ Client safety

DELEGATION

THE CARDIOVASCULAR SYSTEM & THE BLOOD

Level of difficulty: Easy

Overview: This case requires the nurse to identify causes of vitamin B_{12} deficiency, define pernicious anemia, and discuss elements of treatment. Client education is provided regarding preventing injury when experiencing parathesias or peripheral neuropathy.

Client Profile

Mrs. Andersson was diagnosed with pernicious anemia at the age of 70. She has monthly appointments with her primary health care provider for treatment with vitamin B_{12} injections.

Case Study

At the age of 70, Mrs. Andersson was exhibiting weakness, fatigue, and an unexplained weight loss. A complete blood count (CBC) was done as part of her diagnostic workup. The CBC revealed red blood cell count (RBC) 3.20 million/mm^3, mean corpuscular volume (MCV) 130 μL, reticulocytes 0.4%, hematocrit (Hct) 25%, and hemoglobin (Hgb) 7.9 g/dL. Suspecting pernicious anemia, the health care provider prescribed a Shilling test. Mrs. Andersson was diagnosed with pernicious anemia and started on vitamin B_{12} injections.

Questions

1. Briefly describe the pathophysiology of pernicious anemia.

2. Identify possible causes of vitamin B_{12} deficiency.

3. Identify the possible manifestations of pernicious anemia.

4. Identify the physical assessment findings that are characteristic of pernicious anemia.

5. What are the expected results of a complete blood count (CBC) and serum vitamin B_{12} level in a female client with pernicious anemia?

6. How does Mrs. Andersson's ethnicity relate to pernicious anemia?

7. To help make a definitive diagnosis of pernicious anemia, a Schilling test may be performed. Describe the Schilling test.

8. Mrs. Andersson understands that including foods high in vitamin B_{12} in her diet is helpful in preventing vitamin B_{12} deficiency. Identify five foods rich in vitamin B_{12}.

9. Discuss the standard dosing and desired effects of the vitamin B_{12} injections for the client with vitamin B_{12} deficiency.

10. When can Mrs. Andersson discontinue the vitamin B_{12} injections?

11. The nurse administers Mrs. Andersson's vitamin B_{12} injections using the z-track injection method. Discuss why the nurse used this method and the steps of this injection technique.

12. Discuss other possible medications or supplements that may be indicated for the treatment of pernicious anemia.

13. During a routine visit, Mrs. Andersson tells the nurse that she has noticed a decreased sensation in her fingers. "I can pick up a cup, but I can't really feel the cup in my hand. It is a tingling sensation of sorts." What teaching should the nurse initiate to promote Mrs. Andersson's safety at home?

GENDER

Male

AGE

42

SETTING

- Hospital

ETHNICITY

- White American

CULTURAL CONSIDERATIONS

PREEXISTING CONDITIONS

- Pneumonia last year; unexplained fifteen-pound weight loss over past six months

COEXISTING CONDITIONS

- Thrush; pneumonia; human immunodeficiency virus (HIV)

COMMUNICATION

DISABILITY

- Potential disability resulting from chronic illness

SOCIOECONOMIC

- Married for seventeen years; two children (ages 14 and 11 years old); primary income provider for family

SPIRITUAL/RELIGIOUS

PHARMACOLOGIC

LEGAL

- Infectious disease; client confidentiality; partner notification

ETHICAL

- Partner notification of exposure to HIV

ALTERNATIVE THERAPY

PRIORITIZATION

DELEGATION

MODERATE

THE CARDIOVASCULAR SYSTEM & THE BLOOD

Level of difficulty: Moderate

Overview: The nurse in this case is caring for a client who has recently learned that he is positive for the human immunodeficiency virus (HIV). Laboratory testing to monitor the progression of HIV is reviewed. The ethical and legal concerns regarding the client's decision not to disclose his HIV status to his wife or others are discussed.

Client Profile

Mr. Thomas is a 42-year-old man admitted to the hospital with complaints of shortness of breath, fever, fatigue, and oral thrush. The health care provider reviews the laboratory and diagnostic tests with Mr. Thomas and informs him that he has pneumonia and is HIV positive. Mr. Thomas believes that he contracted HIV while involved in an affair with another woman three years ago. He is afraid to tell his wife, knowing she will be angry and that she may leave him.

Case Study

The nurse assigned to care for Mr. Thomas reads in the medical record (chart) that he learned two days ago that he is HIV positive. There is a note in the record that indicates that Mr. Thomas has not told his wife the diagnosis.

To complete a functional health pattern assessment, the nurse asks Mr. Thomas if he may ask him a few questions. Mr. Thomas is willing and in the course of their conversation shares with the nurse that he believes that he contracted the HIV during an affair with another woman. He states, "How can I tell my wife about this? I am so ashamed. It is bad enough that I had an affair, but to have to tell her in this way—I just don't think I can. She is not sick at all. I will just say I have pneumonia and take the medication my health care provider gave me. I do not want my wife or anyone else to know. If she begins to show signs of not feeling well, then I will tell her. I just can't tell anyone. What will people think of me if they know I have AIDS?"

Questions

1. Briefly discuss how HIV is transmitted and how it is not. How can Mr. Thomas prevent the transmission of HIV to his wife and others?

2. Mr. Thomas stated, "What will people think of me if they know I have AIDS?" How can the nurse explain the difference between being HIV positive and having AIDS?

3. Discuss the ethical dilemmas inherent in this case.

4. Does the health care provider have a legal obligation to tell anyone other than Mr. Thomas that he is HIV positive? If so, discuss.

5. Any loss, such as the loss of one's health, results in a grief response. Describe the stages of grief according to Kubler-Ross.

6. Discuss which stage of grief Mr. Thomas is most likely experiencing. Provide examples of Mr. Thomas's behavior that support your decision.

7. What are the laboratory tests used to confirm the diagnosis of HIV infection in an adult?

8. Discuss the function of CD4+ T cells and provide an example of how the CD4+ T-cell count guides the management of HIV.

9. Briefly explain the purpose of viral load blood tests in monitoring the progression of HIV.

10. Mr. Thomas expresses a readiness to learn more about HIV. Discuss the nurse's initial intervention when beginning client teaching, and then discuss the progression of the HIV disease, including an explanation of *primary infection, categories (groups) A, B, and C,* and *four main types of opportunistic infections.*

11. Following the nurse's teaching, Mr. Thomas states, "How stupid I was to have that affair. Not only could it ruin my marriage, but it gave me a death sentence." Share with Mr. Thomas what you know about *long-term survivors, long-term nonprogressors,* and *Highly Active Antiretroviral Therapy (HAART).*

12. Discuss how the nurse should respond if Mr. Thomas's wife approaches him in the hall and asks, "Did the test results come back yet? Do you know what is wrong with my husband?"

13. List five possible nursing diagnoses appropriate to consider for Mr. Thomas.

CASE STUDY 6

Mrs. Darsana

GENDER

Female

AGE

67

SETTING

■ Hospital

ETHNICITY

■ Black American

CULTURAL CONSIDERATIONS

■ Risk of hypertension and heart disease

PREEXISTING CONDITION

■ Hypertension (HTN)

COEXISTING CONDITION

COMMUNICATION

DISABILITY

SOCIOECONOMIC

SPIRITUAL/RELIGIOUS

PHARMACOLOGIC

■ Acetylsalicylic acid (aspirin); enoxaparin (Lovenox); GPIIb/IIIa agents; heparin sodium; morphine sulfate; nitroglycerin; tissue plasminogen activator (tPA)

LEGAL

ETHICAL

ALTERNATIVE THERAPY

PRIORITIZATION

■ Minimizing cardiac damage

DELEGATION

THE CARDIOVASCULAR SYSTEM & THE BLOOD

Level of difficulty: Moderate

Overview: This case requires the nurse to recognize the signs and symptoms of an acute myocardial infarction (MI). The nurse must anticipate appropriate interventions to minimize cardiac damage and preserve myocardial function. Serum laboratory tests and electrocardiogram findings used to diagnose a myocardial infarction are discussed. Criteria to assess when considering reperfusion using a thrombolytic agent are reviewed. The nurse is asked to prioritize the client's nursing diagnoses.

Client Profile

Mrs. Darsana was sitting at a family cookout at approximately 2:00 P.M. when she experienced what she later describes to the nurse as "nausea with some heartburn." Assuming the discomfort was because of something she ate, she dismissed the discomfort and took Tums. After about two hours, she explains, "My heartburn was not much better and it was now more of a dull pain that seemed to spread to my shoulders. I also noticed that I was a little short of breath." Mrs. Darsana told her son what she was feeling. Concerned, her son called emergency medical services.

Case Study

En route to the hospital, emergency medical personnel established an intravenous access. Mrs. Darsana was given four children's chewable aspirins and three sublingual nitroglycerin tablets without relief of her chest pain. She was placed on oxygen 2 liters via nasal cannula. Upon arrival in the emergency department, Mrs. Darsana is very restless. She states, "It feels like an elephant is sitting on my chest." Her vital signs are blood pressure 160/84, pulse 118, respiratory rate 28, and temperature 99.3°F (37.4°C). Her oxygen saturation is 98% on 2 liters of oxygen. A 12-lead electrocardiogram (ECG, EKG) shows sinus tachycardia with a heart rate of 120 beats per minute. An occasional premature ventricular contraction (PVC), T wave inversion, and ST segment elevation are noted. A chest X-ray is within normal limits with no signs of pulmonary edema. Mrs. Darsana's laboratory results include potassium (K^+) 4.0 mEq/L, magnesium (Mg) 1.9 mg/dL, total creatine kinase (CK) 157 μ/L, CK-MB 7.6 ng/mL, relative index 4.8%, and troponin I 2.8 ng/mL. Her stool tests negative for occult blood.

Questions

1. What are the components of the initial nursing assessment of Mrs. Darsana when she arrives in the emergency department?

2. Mrs. Darsana has a history of unstable angina. Explain what this is.

3. Briefly discuss what causes an MI. Include in the discussion the other terms used for this diagnosis.

4. The nurse listens to Mrs. Darsana's heart sounds to see if S_3, S_4, or a murmur can be heard. What would the nurse suspect if these heart sounds were heard?

5. What factors are considered when diagnosing an acute myocardial infarction (AMI)?

6. Besides her unstable angina, what factors increased Mrs. Darsana's risk for an MI?

7. Identify which of Mrs. Darsana's presenting symptoms are consistent with the profile of a client who is having an MI.

8. The nurse overhears Mrs. Darsana's son asking his mother sternly, "Mom. Why didn't you tell me that you were having chest pain sooner? You should have never ignored this. You could have died right there at my house." How might the nurse explain Mrs. Darsana's actions to the son?

9. Provide a rationale for why Mrs. Darsana was given sublingual nitroglycerin and aspirin en route to the hospital.

10. Briefly discuss the laboratory tests that are significant in the determination of an acute myocardial infarction (AMI).

11. Laboratory results follow:

April 1 at 1645:

Total CK = 216 units/L	CK-MB = 5.6 ng/mL	relative index = 2.2%	Troponin I = 2.8 ng/mL

April 2 at 0045:

Total CK = 242 units/L	CK-MB = 8.1 ng/mL	relative index = 3.3%	Troponin I = 5.2 ng/mL

Questions (continued)

April 2 at 0615:

Total CK = 298 units/L   CK-MB = 9.2 ng/mL   relative index = 3.0%   Troponin I = 4.1 ng/mL

April 3 at 0615:

Total CK = 203 units/L   CK-MB = 6.1 ng/mL   relative index = 3.0%   Troponin I = 1.7 ng/mL

Are Mrs. Darsana's laboratory results consistent with those expected for a client having an acute myocardial infarction?

12. Describe four pharmacologic interventions you anticipate will be initiated/considered during an acute MI.

13. Identify five criteria that could exclude an individual as a candidate for thrombolytic therapy with a tissue plasminogen activator (tPA).

14. An echocardiogram reveals that Mrs. Darsana has an ejection fraction of 50%. How could the nurse explain the meaning of this result to Mrs. Darsana?

15. Identify three appropriate nursing diagnoses for the client experiencing an AMI.

16. Rank the following five nursing diagnoses for Mrs. Darsana in priority order.

- Decreased Cardiac Output related to (r/t) ineffective cardiac tissue perfusion secondary to ventricular damage, ischemia, dysrhythmia.
- Deficient Knowledge (condition, treatment, prognosis) r/t lack of exposure, unfamiliarity with information resources.
- Risk for Injury r/t adverse effect of pharmacologic therapy.
- Acute Pain r/t myocardial tissue damage from inadequate blood supply.
- Fear r/t threat to well-being.

Mrs. Yates

GENDER

Female

AGE

70

SETTING

- Home

ETHNICITY

- Black American

CULTURAL CONSIDERATIONS

- The impact of diet on heart failure

PREEXISTING CONDITIONS

- Hypertension (HTN); heart failure (HF, CHF); coronary artery disease (CAD); myocardial infarction (MI) five years ago; ejection fraction (EF) of 55%

COEXISTING CONDITION

COMMUNICATION

DISABILITY

SOCIOECONOMIC

- Widow; lives alone; able to care for self independently; nonsmoker

SPIRITUAL/RELIGIOUS

PHARMACOLOGIC

- Aspirin (acetylsalicylic acid, ASA); clopidogrel bisulfate (Plavix); lisinopril (Prinivil, Zestril); carvedilol (Coreg); furosemide (Lasix); potassium chloride (KCl)

LEGAL

ETHICAL

ALTERNATIVE THERAPY

PRIORITIZATION

DELEGATION

MODERATE

THE CARDIOVASCULAR SYSTEM & THE BLOOD

Level of difficulty: Moderate

Overview: This case requires the nurse to recognize the symptoms of heart failure and collaborate with the primary care provider to initiate treatment. The pathophysiology of heart failure is reviewed. Several heart failure classification systems are defined. Rationales for prescribed diagnostic tests and medications are provided. The nurse must consider the impact of the client's diet on the exacerbation of symptoms and provide teaching. Nursing diagnoses are prioritized to guide care.

Client Profile

Jeraldine Yates is a 70-year-old woman originally from Alabama. She lives alone and is able to manage herself independently. She is active in her community and church. Mrs. Yates was admitted to the hospital two months ago with heart failure. Since her discharge, a visiting nurse visits every other week to assess for symptoms of heart failure and see that Mrs. Yates is continuing to manage well on her own.

Case Study

The visiting nurse stops in to see Mrs. Yates today. The nurse immediately notices that Mrs. Yates's legs are very swollen. Mrs. Yates states, "I noticed they were getting a bit bigger. They are achy, too." The nurse asks Mrs. Yates if she has been weighing herself daily to which Mrs. Yates replies, "I got on that scale the last time you were here, remember?" The nurse weighs Mrs. Yates and she has gained 10 pounds. Additional assessment findings indicate that Mrs. Yates gets short of breath when ambulating from one room to the other (approximately 20 feet) and must sit down to catch her breath. Her oxygen saturation is 95% on room air. Bibasilar crackles are heard when auscultating her lung sounds. The nurse asks Mrs. Yates if she is currently or has in the past few days experienced any chest, arm, or jaw pain or become nauseous or sweaty. Mrs. Yates states, "No, I didn't have any of that. I would know another heart attack. I didn't have one of those." The nurse asks about any back pain, stomach pain, confusion, dizziness, or a feeling that Mrs. Yates might faint. Mrs. Yates denies these symptoms stating, "No. None of that. Just a little more tired than usual lately." Her vital signs are temperature 97.6°F (36.4°C), blood pressure 140/70, pulse 93, and respirations 22. The nurse reviews Mrs. Yates's list of current medications. Mrs. Yates is taking aspirin, clopidogrel bisulfate, lisinopril, and carvedilol. The nurse calls the health care provider who asks the nurse to draw blood for a complete blood count (CBC), basic metabolic panel (BMP), brain natriuretic peptide (B-type natriuretic peptide assay or BNP), troponin, creatine kinase (CPK), creatine kinase-MB (CKMB), and albumin. The health care provider also prescribes oral (PO) furosemide and asks the nurse to arrange an outpatient electrocardiogram (ECG, EKG), chest X-ray, and echocardiogram.

Questions

1. Which assessment findings during the nurse's visit are consistent with heart failure?

2. Why did the visiting nurse ask Mrs. Yates about back pain, stomach pain, confusion, dizziness, or a feeling that she might faint?

3. Discuss anything else the nurse should assess during her visit with Mrs. Yates.

4. Explain what the following terms indicate and include the normal values: *cardiac output, stroke volume, afterload, preload, ejection fraction,* and *central venous pressure.*

5. Discuss the body's compensatory mechanisms during heart failure. Include an explanation of the Frank-Starling law and the neurohormonal model in your discussion.

6. Heart failure can be classified as left or right ventricular failure, systolic versus diastolic, according to the New York Heart Association (NYHA) and using the ACC/AHA (American Heart Association)

guidelines. Explain these four classification systems and the signs and symptoms that characterize each.

7. According to each classification system discussed above in question #6, how would you label the type of heart failure Mrs. Yates is experiencing?

8. Discuss Mrs. Yates's predisposing risk factors for heart failure. Is her age, gender, or ethnicity significant?

9. Provide a rationale for why each of the following medications are included in Mrs. Yates's medication regimen: *aspirin, clopidogrel bisulfate, lisinopril,* and *carvedilol.*

10. The nurse is teaching Mrs. Yates about her newly prescribed furosemide. Explain the rationale for adding furosemide to Mrs. Yates's medication regimen, when she should expect to see the therapeutic results (urination), and instructions regarding the administration of furosemide.

Questions (continued)

11. The visiting nurse asks the primary health care provider if he/she will prescribe potassium chloride for Mrs. Yates. Why has the nurse suggested this?

12. What information will each of the following blood tests provide: *CBC, BMP, BNP, troponin, CPK, CK-MB,* and *albumin*?

13. What will the health care provider look for on the electrocardiogram, chest X-ray, and echocardiogram? What will each diagnostic test tell the physician?

14. Mrs. Yates's son comes to stay with his mother so she will not be alone. What should the nurse tell Mr. Yates about when he should bring his mother to the hospital?

15. The visiting nurse returns the next day. Mrs. Yates does not seem to be diuresing as well as the nurse anticipated. Mrs. Yates is not worse, but the swelling in her legs is still considerable and there is no change in her weight. When asked about her frequency of voiding, Mrs. Yates does not seem to have noticed much difference. While the nurse is unpacking her stethoscope to assess lung sounds, Mrs. Yates says, "Honey, I was just making myself a ham salad sandwich. Would you like one?" The nurse declines and becomes concerned because of this offer. Why is the nurse concerned?

16. The nurse asks Mrs. Yates to tell her more about how she cooks. Specifically, the nurse asks Mrs. Yates about the types of foods and food preparation. With great pride, Mrs. Yates leads the nurse to the kitchen and explains, "Honey. I am from the South and we cook soul food. Today I am cooking my famous pea soup for the church dinner tonight. I use ham hocks. Have you ever had those? My son says they are not good for me. He has been trying to get me to eat healthier foods. Last week he brought me turkey sausage to try instead of my pork sausage in the morning. I know he means well but some foods are tradition and you don't break soul food tradition." What information has the nurse gathered that is of concern?

17. The nurse arranges for Mrs. Yates's son to be present at the next home visit so that the nurse can teach them both about proper dietary choices and fluid restrictions. List five points of information that the nurse should include in the teaching.

18. During the dietary teaching, the nurse asks Mrs. Yates to describe a typical day of meals and snacks. Mrs. Yates lists coffee with whole milk, eggs and sausage for breakfast, a sandwich or soup for lunch, fried chicken with vegetables for dinner, and fruit, pretzels, or rice pudding for snacks. Which of these foods will the nurse instruct Mrs. Yates to limit and are there alternatives that the nurse can suggest?

19. Since changing her diet, Mrs. Yates has responded to her outpatient treatment plan and has noticed marked improvement in how she feels. The nurse wants to make sure that Mrs. Yates understands the importance of monitoring her weight. What instructions should the nurse give Mrs. Yates regarding how often to weigh herself, and what weight change should be reported to her health care provider or the nurse?

20. Prioritize five nursing diagnoses that the visiting nurse should consider for the recent events regarding Mrs. Yates's care.

Ms. Fox

GENDER

Female

AGE

20

SETTING

- Hospital

ETHNICITY

- Black American

CULTURAL CONSIDERATIONS

- Increased risk for sickle cell disease

PREEXISTING CONDITION

- Sickle cell disease

COEXISTING CONDITION

COMMUNICATION

DISABILITY

SOCIOECONOMIC

- Risk for substance abuse

SPIRITUAL/RELIGIOUS

PHARMACOLOGIC

- Acetaminophen (Tylenol); hydroxyurea (Droxia); morphine sulfate (MS contin); ibuprofen (Advil, Motrin); acetaminophen 300 mg/codeine 30 mg (Tylenol with codeine No. 3); meperidine hydrochloride (Demerol); hydromorphone hydrochloride (Dilaudid)

LEGAL

ETHICAL

ALTERNATIVE THERAPY

- Breathing techniques; relaxation; distraction; transcutaneous nerve stimulation (TENS)

PRIORITIZATION

DELEGATION

THE CARDIOVASCULAR SYSTEM & THE BLOOD

Level of difficulty: Difficult

Overview: This case requires the nurse to define different types of anemia, recognize the symptoms of a sickle cell crisis, and discuss short- and long-term management of sickle cell disease. Nursing diagnoses appropriate for the client are prioritized.

DIFFICULT

Client Profile   **Ms. Fox** is a 20-year-old black American who presents to the emergency department with complaints of chest pain and some shortness of breath. Ms. Fox indicates that she has had a nonproductive cough and low-grade fever for the past two days. She recognizes these symptoms as typical of her sickle cell crisis episodes and knew it was important she come in to get treatment.

Case Study   Ms. Fox was diagnosed with sickle cell anemia as a child and has had multiple crises requiring hospitalization. Ms. Fox states that the pain in her chest is an "8" on a 0 to 10 pain scale. She describes the pain as a "constant burning pain." Her vital signs are temperature of 100.8°F (38.2°C), blood pressure 120/76, pulse 96, and respiratory rate of 22. Her oxygen saturation on room air is 94%. She is having some difficulty breathing and is placed on 2 liters of oxygen by nasal cannula. Ms. Fox explains that she took Extra Strength Tylenol for the past two days in an effort to manage the pain, but when this did not work and the pain got worse, she came in for a stronger pain medication. She explains that in the past she has been given morphine for the pain and prefers to use the patient-controlled analgesia (PCA) pump. Blood work reveals the following values: white blood cell count (WBC) 18,000 cells/mm^3, red blood cell count (RBC) 3×10^6, mean corpuscular volume (MCV) 70 μm^3, red cell distribution width (RDW) 20.4%, hemoglobin (Hgb) 7.5 g/dL, hematocrit (Hct) 21.8%, and reticulocyte count 23%. Ms. Fox is admitted for pain management, antibiotic treatment, and respiratory support.

Questions

1. Three types of anemia are *hypoproliferative, bleeding,* and *hemolytic.* Provide a basic definition of the etiology of each type and one example of each type.

2. Discuss how Ms. Fox's laboratory results are consistent with clients who have sickle cell anemia.

3. Describe the structure and function of normal red blood cells in the body.

4. Describe the structure and effects of red blood cells (RBCs) that contain sickle cell hemoglobin molecules.

5. Is sickle cell anemia an inherited anemia or an acquired anemia? Explain.

6. Discuss the relationship between sickle cell anemia and Ms. Fox's ethnicity.

7. Discuss the characteristic signs and symptoms of sickle cell anemia.

8. Discuss the potential complications associated with sickle cell anemia.

9. Describe the pharmacologic management for a client with sickle cell anemia. Include a discussion of the potential adverse effects of the medication.

10. Describe the use of transfusion therapy for management of sickle cell anemia. Include a discussion of the potential complications of chronic red blood cell transfusions.

11. Bone marrow transplantation (BMT) offers a potential cure for sickle cell disease. Why is BMT a treatment option available to only a small number of clients with sickle cell disease?

12. In the adult, three types of sickle cell crisis are possible: sickle crisis, aplastic crisis, and sequestration crisis. Briefly describe the pathophysiological changes that lead to each type.

13. There are four common patterns of an acute vaso-occlusive sickle cell crisis: *bone crisis, acute chest syndrome, abdominal crisis,* and *joint crisis.* Briefly describe the characteristic symptoms of each pattern.

14. Which pattern discussed in question number 13 is most congruent with Ms. Fox's presenting signs and symptoms?

15. Discuss the symptoms the nurse should look for while completing an assessment of a client in potential sickle cell (vaso-occlusive) crisis.

16. Briefly discuss the factors that can trigger a sickle cell crisis.

17. Prioritize three potential nursing diagnoses appropriate for Ms. Fox.

18. Describe the nursing management goals during the acute phase of a sickle cell crisis.

19. Explain why individuals with sickle cell disease may be at risk for substance abuse.

20. Discuss the long-term prognosis for Ms. Fox.

Mrs. O'Grady

GENDER

Female

AGE

55

SETTING

- Hospital

ETHNICITY

- White American

CULTURAL CONSIDERATIONS

PREEXISTING CONDITIONS

- Hypertension (HTN); angina; total abdominal hysterectomy six months ago; allergy to shellfish

COEXISTING CONDITION

- Positive myocardial perfusion imaging study (stress test)

COMMUNICATION

DISABILITY

SOCIOECONOMIC

SPIRITUAL/RELIGIOUS

PHARMACOLOGIC

- Dipyridamole (Persantine); atenolol (Tenormin); atorvastatin calcium (Lipitor); conjugated estrogen, oral (Premarin)

LEGAL

- Informed consent

ETHICAL

ALTERNATIVE THERAPY

PRIORITIZATION

DELEGATION

THE CARDIOVASCULAR SYSTEM & THE BLOOD

Level of difficulty: Difficult

Overview: This case requires the nurse to convey an understanding of the cardiac catheterization procedure. Appropriate client care pre- and postcardiac catheterization is discussed. The client's current medications are reviewed. Discharge teaching is provided.

DIFFICULT

Client Profile

Mrs. O'Grady is a 55-year-old female with a history of angina and recent hospital admission for complaints of chest pain and shortness of breath. It is determined that she did not suffer a myocardial infarction. Mrs. O'Grady's health care provider has scheduled her for a cardiac catheterization after learning that the results of her dipyridamole (Persantine) myocardial perfusion imaging study (stress test) were abnormal.

Case Study

Mrs. O'Grady is having a cardiac catheterization today. The cardiac catheterization lab nurse assigned to care for Mrs. O'Grady will provide teaching, check to see that there are no contraindications for Mrs. O'Grady consenting to the procedure, and provide pre- and postprocedure care.

Questions

1. Why has Mrs. O'Grady's health care provider prescribed a cardiac catheterization? What information will this procedure provide?

2. What are the potential contraindications that can prevent someone from being able to have a cardiac catheterization? What is the contraindication that must be considered in Mrs. O'Grady's case? Why is this of concern?

3. Discuss the preprocedure assessments the nurse will complete prior to Mrs. O'Grady's cardiac catheterization.

4. Discuss interventions the nurse will complete prior to Mrs. O'Grady's cardiac catheterization.

5. Provide a brief rationale for why each of the following medications have been prescribed for Mrs. O'Grady: atenolol (Tenormin); atorvastatin calcium (Lipitor); conjugated estrogen, oral (Premarin).

6. What are two appropriate nursing diagnoses to consider for Mrs. O'Grady prior to her having the cardiac catheterization?

7. Mrs. O'Grady asks the nurse, "What are they going to do to me today?" Explain what a cardiac catheterization involves and how long Mrs. O'Grady can expect the procedure to last. Briefly describe the difference between a left-sided and right-sided catheterization.

8. What are the risks of having a cardiac catheterization? What are the two most common complications during the procedure?

9. List at least five manifestations of an adverse reaction to the contrast dye the nurse will watch for.

10. How should the nurse respond when Mrs. O'Grady asks, "How soon will I know if something is wrong with me?"

11. What is "informed consent"? Is consent required prior to a cardiac catheterization? Why or why not?

12. Immediately following the cardiac catheterization procedure, what is the nurse's responsibility to help minimize bleeding at the femoral puncture site, and what will be Mrs. O'Grady's prescribed activity?

13. Discuss the priorities of the nursing assessment following a femoral cardiac catheterization. Be sure to note in your discussion when the health care provider should be notified.

14. What are two nursing diagnoses to consider for Mrs. O'Grady following the cardiac catheterization?

15. Mrs. O'Grady has a left groin puncture site. She needs to go to the bathroom, but is still on bed rest. What is the proper way for the nurse to assist her?

16. The results of Mrs. O'Grady's cardiac catheterization indicate that she does not have any significant heart disease and her coronary arteries are patent. The health care provider discharges her. Her husband has been called to bring her home. What instructions should the nurse provide regarding activity, diet, and medications?

PART TWO

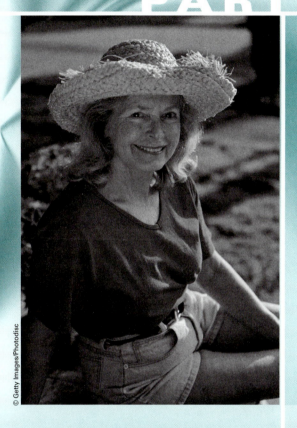

The Respiratory System

CASE STUDY 1

Mrs. Hogan

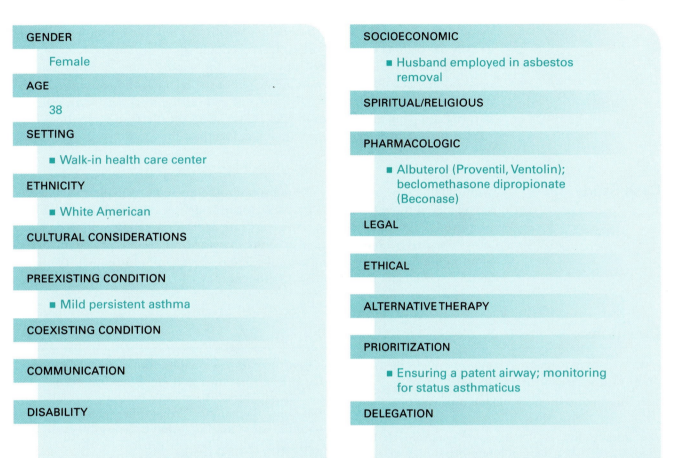

GENDER

Female

AGE

38

SETTING

■ Walk-in health care center

ETHNICITY

■ White American

CULTURAL CONSIDERATIONS

PREEXISTING CONDITION

■ Mild persistent asthma

COEXISTING CONDITION

COMMUNICATION

DISABILITY

SOCIOECONOMIC

■ Husband employed in asbestos removal

SPIRITUAL/RELIGIOUS

PHARMACOLOGIC

■ Albuterol (Proventil, Ventolin); beclomethasone dipropionate (Beconase)

LEGAL

ETHICAL

ALTERNATIVE THERAPY

PRIORITIZATION

■ Ensuring a patent airway; monitoring for status asthmaticus

DELEGATION

THE RESPIRATORY SYSTEM

Level of difficulty: Easy

Overview: This case requires that the nurse recognize appropriate interventions for an asthma attack and understand the actions of respiratory medications. The nurse must assess the triggers specific to this patient and provide teaching to reduce the patient's risk of another exacerbation. Priority nursing diagnoses and outcome goals are identified.

Client Profile

Mrs. Hogan is a 38-year-old woman brought to a walk-in health care center by her neighbor. Mrs. Hogan is in obvious respiratory distress. She is having difficulty breathing with audible high-pitched wheezing and is having difficulty speaking. Pausing after every few words to catch her breath, she tells the nurse, "I am having a really bad asthma attack. My chest feels very tight and I cannot catch my breath. I took my albuterol and Vanceril, but they are not helping." Mrs. Hogan hands her neighbor her cell phone and asks the neighbor to dial a telephone number. "That number is my husband's boss. My husband just started working for an asbestos removal company about a month ago. He is usually on the road somewhere. Can you ask his boss to get a message to him that I am here?"

Case Study

While auscultating Mrs. Hogan's lung sounds, the nurse hears expiratory wheezes and scattered rhonchi throughout. Mrs. Hogan is afebrile. Her vital signs are blood pressure 142/96, pulse 88, and respiratory rate 34. Her oxygen saturation on room air is 86%. Arterial blood gases (ABGs) are drawn. Mrs. Hogan is placed on 2 liters of humidified oxygen via nasal cannula. She is started on intravenous (IV) fluids and receives an albuterol nebulizer treatment.

Questions

1. What other signs and symptoms might the nurse note during assessment of Mrs. Hogan?

2. In what position should the nurse place Mrs. Hogan and why?

3. Identify at least five signs and symptoms that indicate that Mrs. Hogan is not responding to treatment and may be developing status asthmaticus (a life-threatening condition).

4. Mrs. Hogan states that she took her albuterol and beclomethasone prior to coming to the walk-in health care center. How do these medications work?

5. Briefly discuss the common adverse effects Mrs. Hogan may experience with the albuterol nebulizer treatment.

6. Physiologically, what is happening in Mrs. Hogan's lungs during an asthma attack?

7. In order of priority, identify three nursing diagnoses that are appropriate during Mrs. Hogan's asthma exacerbation.

8. Write three outcome goals for Mrs. Hogan's diagnosis of Ineffective Breathing Pattern.

9. Mrs. Hogan has responded well to the albuterol nebulizer treatment. Her breathing is less labored and she appears less anxious. The nurse asks Mrs. Hogan what she was doing when the asthma attack began. Mrs. Hogan says, "Nothing special. I was doing the laundry." What other questions might the nurse ask (and why) to assess the cause of Mrs. Hogan's asthma exacerbation?

10. What are some other questions the nurse might ask to get a better sense of Mrs. Hogan's asthma?

11. The nurse asks Mrs. Hogan to describe step-by-step how she uses her inhalers. Mrs. Hogan describes the following steps: "First I shake the inhaler well. Then I breathe out normally and place the mouthpiece in my mouth. I take a few breaths and then while breathing in slowly and deeply with my lips tight around the mouthpiece, I give myself a puff. I hold my breath for a count of five and breathe out slowly as if I am blowing out a candle. I wait a minute or two and then I repeat those steps all over again for my second puff." Which step(s) is/are of concern to the nurse and why?

12. Briefly discuss three nursing interventions to help decrease Mrs. Hogan's risk of another asthma exacerbation.

William

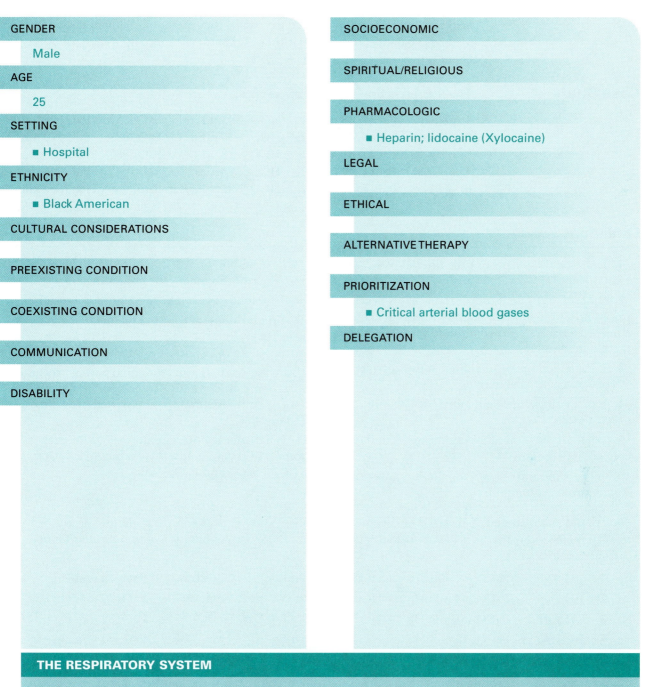

EASY

GENDER

Male

AGE

25

SETTING

■ Hospital

ETHNICITY

■ Black American

CULTURAL CONSIDERATIONS

PREEXISTING CONDITION

COEXISTING CONDITION

COMMUNICATION

DISABILITY

SOCIOECONOMIC

SPIRITUAL/RELIGIOUS

PHARMACOLOGIC

■ Heparin; lidocaine (Xylocaine)

LEGAL

ETHICAL

ALTERNATIVE THERAPY

PRIORITIZATION

■ Critical arterial blood gases

DELEGATION

THE RESPIRATORY SYSTEM

Level of difficulty: Easy

Overview: This case provides the nurse with an opportunity to convey an understanding of the arterial blood gas testing method and practice the skill of acid-base analysis/arterial blood gas results interpretation.

Client Profile   **William** is a newly graduated registered nurse. He will begin working on a respiratory nursing unit next week. During orientation to his role, he will learn how to collect an arterial blood gas (ABG) sample. He is given five sets of ABG results to practice acid-base analysis/arterial blood gas results interpretation. William must determine acid-base balance, determine if there is compensation, and decide whether each client is hypoxic.

Case Study   The five sets of arterial blood gas results are:

1. pH 6.95 $PaCO_2$ 48 mm Hg HCO_3^- 23 mEq/L SaO_2 95% PaO_2 79 mm Hg
2. pH 7.48 $PaCO_2$ 44 mm Hg HCO_3^- 30 mEq/L SaO_2 88% PaO_2 70 mm Hg
3. pH 7.48 $PaCO_2$ 31 mm Hg HCO_3^- 19 mEq/L SaO_2 93% PaO_2 82 mm Hg
4. pH 7.35 $PaCO_2$ 42 mm Hg HCO_3^- 26 mEq/L SaO_2 95% PaO_2 83 mm Hg
5. pH 7.53 $PaCO_2$ 31 mm Hg HCO_3^- 35 mEq/L SaO_2 90% PaO_2 57 mm Hg

Questions

1. Describe the purpose of the arterial blood gas (ABG) test.

2. Describe the client preparation that is necessary prior to drawing an ABG sample. Is written client consent (a consent form) required prior to drawing the blood sample?

3. List the equipment the nurse must gather prior to collecting the ABG sample.

4. List the steps for obtaining an ABG sample from a radial artery.

5. What are the potential complications of the ABG collection procedure?

6. Discuss the nursing responsibilities after the ABG sample is obtained.

7. Explain how an ABG sample should be transported to the laboratory for processing.

8. How long does it take to obtain ABG results?

9. Briefly discuss at least five factors that can cause false ABG results.

10. What are the normal ranges for each of the ABG components in an adult: pH, partial pressure of carbon dioxide ($PaCO_2$), bicarbonate (HCO_3^-), oxygen saturation (SaO_2), and partial pressure of oxygen (PaO_2)?

11. What are the critical/panic values for each of the ABG components in an adult: pH, $PaCO_2$, HCO_3^-, SaO_2, and PaO_2?

12. Help William analyze each set of ABG results. Determine whether each value is high, low, or within normal limits; interpret the acid-base balance; determine if there is compensation; and indicate whether the client is hypoxic.

1. pH 6.95 $PaCO_2$ 48 mm Hg HCO_3^- 23 mEq/L SaO_2 95% PaO_2 79 mm Hg
2. pH 7.48 $PaCO_2$ 44 mm Hg HCO_3^- 30 mEq/L SaO_2 88% PaO_2 70 mm Hg
3. pH 7.48 $PaCO_2$ 31 mm Hg HCO_3^- 19 mEq/L SaO_2 93% PaO_2 82 mm Hg
4. pH 7.35 $PaCO_2$ 42 mm Hg HCO_3^- 26 mEq/L SaO_2 96% PaO_2 83 mm Hg
5. pH 7.53 $PaCO_2$ 31 mm Hg HCO_3^- 35 mEq/L SaO_2 90% PaO_2 57 mm Hg

13. Identify three appropriate nursing diagnoses for a client having an ABG sample obtained.

MODERATE

GENDER

Male

AGE

75

SETTING

- Hospital

ETHNICITY

- Jewish American

CULTURAL CONSIDERATIONS

- Perception and expression of pain

PREEXISTING CONDITIONS

- Chronic obstructive pulmonary disease (COPD) (emphysema); hypertension (HTN) well controlled by enalapril (Vasotec)

COEXISTING CONDITION

- Lower back pain

COMMUNICATION

DISABILITY

- Needs assistance of one person while ambulating due to unsteady gait and dyspnea on exertion

SOCIOECONOMIC

SPIRITUAL/RELIGIOUS

- Judaism

PHARMACOLOGIC

- Acetaminophen (Tylenol); albuterol (AccuNeb, Proventil, Ventolin); enalapril (Vasotec); oxycodone/ acetaminophen (Percocet)

LEGAL

ETHICAL

ALTERNATIVE THERAPY

- Nonpharmacologic interventions for respiratory distress and pain management

PRIORITIZATION

- Difficulty breathing; pain management

DELEGATION

THE RESPIRATORY SYSTEM

Level of difficulty: Moderate

Overview: This case requires that the nurse recognize the signs and symptoms of activity intolerance and respiratory distress and how symptoms differ in the client who has COPD. The nurse considers both pharmacologic and nonpharmacologic interventions to manage respiratory distress and pain. Cultural/spiritual perceptions of pain and pain management are discussed. The nurse must provide discharge teaching regarding safe use of oxygen in the home.

Client Profile

Mr. Cohen is a 75-year-old male admitted with an exacerbation of chronic obstructive pulmonary disease (emphysema). He has been keeping the head of the bed up for most of the day and night to facilitate his breathing which has resulted in lower back pain. Acetaminophen (Tylenol) was not effective in reducing his pain, so the health care provider has prescribed oxycodone/acetaminophen (Percocet) one to two tablets PO every four to six hours as needed for pain. Mr. Cohen is on 2 liters of oxygen by nasal cannula. He can receive respiratory treatments of albuterol (AccuNeb, Proventil, Ventolin) every six hours as needed. Mr. Cohen needs someone to walk beside him when he ambulates because he has an unsteady gait and often needs to stop to catch his breath.

Case Study

The nurse enters the room and finds Mr. Cohen hunched over his bedside table watching television. He says this position helps his breathing. His lung sounds are clear but diminished bilaterally. Capillary refill is four seconds and slight clubbing of his fingers is noted. His oxygen saturation is being assessed every two hours to monitor for hypoxia. Each assessment reveals oxygen saturation at rest of 90% to 94% on 2 liters of oxygen by nasal cannula.

After breakfast, Mr. Cohen complains of lower back pain that caused him increased discomfort while ambulating to the bathroom. He describes the pain as a dull ache and rates the pain a "6" on a 0–10 pain scale. He requests two Percocet tablets. The nurse assesses Mr. Cohen's vital signs (blood pressure 150/78, pulse 90, respiratory rate 26) and gives the Percocet as prescribed. Forty-five minutes later, Mr. Cohen states the Percocet has helped relieve his back pain to a "2" on a 0–10 pain scale and he would like to take a walk in the hall. The nurse checks his oxygen saturation before they leave his room, and it is 92%. Using a portable oxygen tank, the nurse walks with Mr. Cohen from his room to the nurse's station (approximately 60 feet). Mr. Cohen stops to rest at the nurse's station because he is short of breath. His oxygen saturation at the nurse's station is 86%. After a few deep breaths and rest, his oxygen saturation rises to 91%. Mr. Cohen walks back to his room where he sits in his recliner to wait for lunch. His oxygen saturation is initially 87% when he returns and then 91% after a few minutes of rest. Expiratory wheezes are heard bilaterally when the nurse assesses his lung sounds. While Mr. Cohen waits for lunch to arrive, the nurse calls respiratory therapy to give Mr. Cohen his albuterol treatment. The respiratory treatment and rest relieves his acute shortness of breath. His oxygen saturation is now 93%, and his lung sounds are clear but diminished bilaterally.

Questions

1. Briefly define chronic obstructive pulmonary disease (COPD). What pathophysiology is occurring in the lungs of a client with emphysema?

2. What are five signs and symptoms of respiratory distress the nurse may observe in a client with COPD?

3. Describe the physical appearance characteristics of a client with emphysema.

4. Are Mr. Cohen's oxygen saturation readings normal? Explain your answer.

5. Explain the effects that acute pain can have on an individual's respiratory pattern and cardiovascular system.

6. List five nonpharmacologic interventions that the nurse could implement to help decrease Mr. Cohen's difficulty breathing.

7. How would the nurse measure the effectiveness of the interventions suggested in question number 6?

8. Explain why the nurse did not increase Mr. Cohen's oxygen to help ease his shortness of breath.

Questions (continued)

9. Discuss the cultural/spiritual considerations the nurse should keep in mind while creating a plan of care for Mr. Cohen's pain management.

10. What are three nonpharmacologic nursing interventions to help manage Mr. Cohen's pain?

11. How would the nurse measure the effectiveness of the interventions suggested in question number 10?

12. Should the nurse be concerned about the adverse effects of respiratory depression and hypotension when giving oxycodone/acetaminophen (Percocet) to Mr. Cohen? Why or why not?

13. What are three nursing diagnoses that address physical and/or physiological safety concerns for Mr. Cohen?

14. Mr. Cohen will be returning home with oxygen. List at least five safety considerations the nurse should include in discharge teaching regarding the use of oxygen in the home.

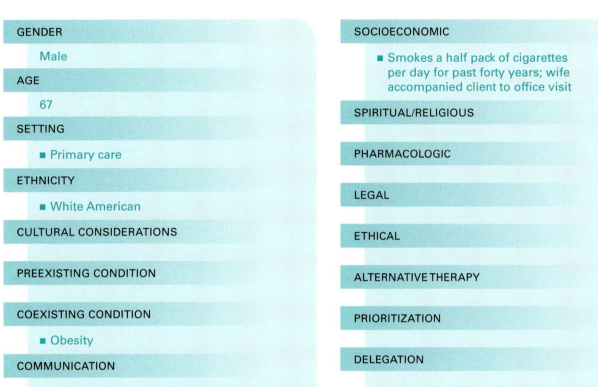

GENDER	**SOCIOECONOMIC**
Male	■ Smokes a half pack of cigarettes per day for past forty years; wife accompanied client to office visit
AGE	
67	
	SPIRITUAL/RELIGIOUS
SETTING	
■ Primary care	**PHARMACOLOGIC**
ETHNICITY	
■ White American	**LEGAL**
CULTURAL CONSIDERATIONS	
	ETHICAL
PREEXISTING CONDITION	
	ALTERNATIVE THERAPY
COEXISTING CONDITION	
■ Obesity	**PRIORITIZATION**
COMMUNICATION	
	DELEGATION
DISABILITY	

MODERATE

THE RESPIRATORY SYSTEM

Level of difficulty: Moderate

Overview: This case reviews the normal sleep cycle of an adult. The nurse must identify the symptoms of sleep apnea syndrome. Potential long-term complications of obstructive sleep apnea syndrome are discussed and treatment options are considered.

Client Profile

Mr. Kaberry is a 67-year-old man. He is 5 feet, 10 inches tall. Over the past five years, Mr. Kaberry has gained 50 pounds and currently weighs 260 pounds (118.2 kg). He smokes a half pack of cigarettes each day and has been a smoker for the past forty years. In the past three months, he has noticed that, despite sleeping for at least seven hours a night, he is very tired during the day. He is afraid he is ill and has made an appointment with his primary health care provider.

Case Study

While conducting an initial assessment, the nurse asks Mr. Kaberry what brought him to the provider's office. Mr. Kaberry states, "I have been so tired during the day. I realize I have put on weight over the last few years, but I am so exhausted. I work in a bank and sometimes I wish I could just put my head on my desk at and catch a quick nap. That is not like me. I usually feel rested in the morning and I never take naps during the day. There must be something wrong with me." Mrs. Kaberry adds, "If anyone should be tired it is me. He keeps me up most of the night with his snoring. I hope you can find out what is wrong with him because living with him has been unbearable lately." The nurse asks Mrs. Kaberry to explain what she means by "unbearable." Mrs. Kaberry explains that Mr. Kaberry has been short with her, "Very irritable, I guess you could say."

Questions

1. Describe the five stages of sleep and the normal sleep cycle of an adult.

2. How is sleep apnea syndrome defined and what are the three types of sleep apnea?

3. How does Mr. Kaberry fit the profile of the "typical" client who has sleep apnea?

4. The nurse continues the assessment of Mr. Kaberry's symptoms. List at least five other manifestations of sleep apnea the nurse should ask if he has experienced.

5. Briefly discuss Mr. Kaberry's predisposing risk factors for sleep apnea syndrome. How common is sleep apnea in the United States?

6. Discuss the anatomy and physiology that causes obstructive sleep apnea syndrome.

7. Explain how sleep apnea syndrome is diagnosed.

8. What are the potential complications associated with sleep apnea syndrome?

9. Discuss the interventions to consider when planning the medical management of Mr. Kaberry's obstructive sleep apnea. Include a discussion of positive airway pressure therapy.

10. How will the nurse respond when Mrs. Kaberry asks "Do we really need that machine? Isn't there a medication he could take to help this problem?"

11. Mr. and Mrs. Kaberry are learning how to use the CPAP machine. What are two potential side effects experienced by people using CPAP therapy and what are two interventions that can help decrease the side effects?

12. When teaching Mr. and Mrs. Kaberry how to use the CPAP machine, what relationship and body image concerns should be acknowledged?

13. Surgery may be an option for Mr. Kaberry if the symptoms of his obstructive sleep apnea do not improve with nonsurgical interventions. What surgical procedures are used to treat obstructive sleep apnea?

14. Help the nurse generate three appropriate nursing diagnoses for Mr. Kaberry.

15. Until Mr. Kaberry's sleep apnea responds to treatment and his fatigue resolves, what safety precaution(s) should the nurse suggest?

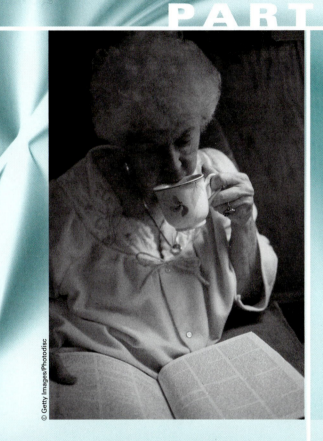

The Nervous/ Neurological System

GENDER

Female

AGE

43

SETTING

- Emergency department

ETHNICITY

- White American

CULTURAL CONSIDERATIONS

PREEXISTING CONDITION

COEXISTING CONDITION

- Herpes Simplex virus type 1

COMMUNICATION

DISABILITY

SOCIOECONOMIC

- Married

SPIRITUAL/RELIGIOUS

PHARMACOLOGIC

- Acyclovir; Prednisone

LEGAL

ETHICAL

ALTERNATIVE THERAPY

- Acupuncture

PRIORITIZATION

DELEGATION

THE NERVOUS/NEUROLOGICAL SYSTEM

Level of difficulty: Easy

Overview: This case requires the nurse to discuss Bell's palsy. An understanding of pharmacological treatments and cranial nerve testing is needed. Nursing diagnoses for priority care are identified.

Client Profile

Mrs. Seaborn is a 43-year-old woman who presents to the emergency department with complaints of weakness of the left side of her face. She is married and is an interior decorator who owns her own business. Earlier today she was working at a client's home when she started to have increased facial weakness and was unable to taste her lunch. She states a history of two days of numbness in her forehead.

Case Study

Mrs. Seaborn's vital signs are temperature 98.2°F, blood pressure 148/60, pulse 83, and respiratory rate of 26. She is fearful, crying, and states, "My mother died of a stroke, I am sure that is what is going on. Am I going to die?" She complains of pain behind and in front of her left ear. She is exhibiting unilateral facial paralysis. Her left eye is drooping and she says it feels dry. Her inability to raise her eyebrow, puff out her cheeks, frown, smile or wrinkle her forehead is suspicious for Bell's palsy. A healing cold sore is observed on her lower lip.

Questions

1. Define Bell's palsy and identify two conditions that could mimic it.

2. What is the main cranial nerve involved with Bell's palsy? How is testing done for this nerve?

3. What significance does Mrs. Seaborn's current cold sore on her lip have with Bell's palsy?

4. What other tests may be needed to rule out other causes of Bell's palsy?

5. What other symptoms would you expect to occur for Mrs. Seaborn?

6. What are three priority nursing diagnoses for Mrs. Seaborn?

7. Discuss the nonsurgical management for Bell's palsy.

8. Discuss further complications of Bell's palsy.

9. What is the normal expected recovery time for Mrs. Seaborn?

Mrs. Giammo

GENDER

Female

AGE

59

SETTING

- Hospital

ETHNICITY

- Black American

CULTURAL CONSIDERATIONS

PREEXISTING CONDITION

- Hypertension (HTN)

COEXISTING CONDITION

- Hypercholesterolemia

COMMUNICATION

DISABILITY

SOCIOECONOMIC

- History of tobacco use for twenty-five years—quit ten years ago; husband smokes one pack per day; positive family history of heart disease; occasionally takes walks in the neighborhood with friends but does not have a regular exercise regimen

SPIRITUAL/RELIGIOUS

PHARMACOLOGIC

- Atenolol (Tenormin); heparin (Heparin Sodium); atorvastatin (Lipitor)

LEGAL

ETHICAL

ALTERNATIVE THERAPY

- Lifestyle modification

PRIORITIZATION

DELEGATION

THE NERVOUS/NEUROLOGICAL SYSTEM

Level of difficulty: Easy

Overview: This case requires the nurse to recognize the signs and symptoms of a transient ischemic attack (TIA) and define the difference between a cerebrovascular accident (CVA, stroke) and a TIA. The nurse must recognize the risk factors for a possible stroke and suggest lifestyle modifications to decrease risk. Explanations of test results and physical assessment findings are offered. Appropriate nursing diagnoses for this client are prioritized.

Client Profile

Mrs. Giammo is a 59-year-old woman who was brought to the emergency department by her husband. Mr. Giammo noticed that all of a sudden his wife "was slurring her speech and her face was drooping on one side." Mrs. Giammo told her husband that she felt some numbness on the right side of her face and in her right arm. Mr. Giammo was afraid his wife was having a stroke so he brought her to the hospital.

Case Study

In the emergency department, Mrs. Giammo is alert and oriented. Her vital signs are temperature 98.2°F (36.7°C), blood pressure 148/97, pulse 81, and respiratory rate 14. An electrocardiogram (ECG, EKG) monitor shows a normal sinus rhythm. Mrs. Giammo is still complaining of "numbness" of the right side of her face and down her right arm. Her mouth is noted to divert to the right side with a slight facial droop when she smiles. Her speech is clear. She is able to move all of her extremities and follow commands. Her pupils are round, equal, and reactive to light (4 mm to 2 mm) and accommodation. There is no nystagmus noted. Her right hand grasp is weaker than her left. Mrs. Giammo does not have a headache and denies any nausea, vomiting, chest pain, diaphoresis, or visual complaints. She is not experiencing any significant weakness, has a steady gait, and is able to swallow without difficulty. Laboratory blood test results are as follows: white blood cell count (WBC) 8,000 cells/mm^3, hemoglobin (Hgb) 14 g/dL, hematocrit (Hct) 44%, platelets = 294,000 mm^3, erythrocyte sedimentation rate (ESR) 15 mm/hr, prothrombin time (PT) 12.9 seconds, international normalized ratio (INR) 1.10, sodium (Na^{2+}) 149 mEq/L, potassium (K$^+$) 4.5 mEq/L, glucose 105 mg/dL, calcium (Ca^{2+}) 9.5 mg/dL, blood urea nitrogen (BUN) 15 mg/dL, and creatinine (creat) 0.8 mg/dL. A head computed tomography (CT) scan is done which shows no acute intracranial change and a magnetic resonance imagery (MRI) is within normal limits. Mrs. Giammo is started on an intravenous heparin drip of 25,000 units in 500 cc of D5W at 18 mL per hour (900 units per hour). Mrs. Giammo is admitted for a neurology evaluation, magnetic resonance angiography (MRA) of the brain, a fasting serum cholesterol, and blood pressure monitoring. Upon admission to the nursing unit, her symptoms have resolved. There is no facial asymmetry and her complaint of numbness has subsided.

Questions

1. The neurologist's consult report states, "At no time during the episode of numbness did the client ever develop any scotoma, amaurosis, ataxia, or diplopia." Explain what these terms mean.

2. The neurology consult report includes the following statement: "Client's diet is notable for moderate amounts of aspartame and no significant glutamate." What are *aspartame* and *glutamate*? Why did the neurologist assess Mrs. Giammo's intake of aspartame and glutamate?

3. Discuss the pathophysiology of a transient ischemic attack (TIA). Include in your discussion what causes a TIA and the natural course of a TIA.

4. Mrs. Giammo asks, "How is what I had different from a stroke?" Provide a simple explanation of how a transient ischemic attack (TIA) differs from a cerebrovascular accident (CVA, stroke).

5. Discuss the defining characteristics of a transient ischemic attack (TIA).

6. How does Mrs. Giammo's case fit the profile of the "typical" client with a TIA?

7. Mrs. Giammo has her fasting cholesterol levels checked. How long must Mrs. Giammo fast before the test?

8. Mrs. Giammo's cholesterol lab work reveals total cholesterol = 242 mg/dL, low-density lipoprotein (LDL) = 165 mg/dL, high-density lipoprotein (HDL) = 30 mg/dL. Discuss the normal values of each and which of her results are of concern and why.

Questions (continued)

9. When told that her cholesterol levels are elevated, Mrs. Giammo asks, "I always see commercials on television saying you should lower your cholesterol. What is cholesterol anyway?" How could the nurse explain what cholesterol is and why it increases the risk of heart disease and stroke?

10. Identify Mrs. Giammo's predisposing risk factors for a TIA and possible stroke. Which factors can she change and which factors are beyond her control?

11. Mrs. Giammo takes atenolol at home. What is the most likely reason why she has been prescribed this medication?

12. The nurse hears a carotid bruit on physical assessment. What is a bruit and why is this of concern to the nurse? What would be likely diagnostic procedures ordered by the health care provider because of this assessment finding?

13. If a carotid ultrasound, carotid duplex, and/or MRA reveals carotid artery stenosis, what surgical procedure can resolve the stenosis?

14. Provide a simple rationale for including intravenous heparin in Mrs. Giammo's treatment plan.

15. Identify the potential life-threatening adverse effects/complications of heparin therapy and the treatment of heparin toxicity or overdose.

16. To assess for bleeding and possible hemorrhage, explain what the nurse monitors while Mrs. Giammo is on heparin therapy.

17. What is the major complication associated with a TIA?

18. Identify six nursing diagnoses in order of priority appropriate for Mrs. Giammo.

19. Atorvastatin 10 mg PO per day is prescribed for Mrs. Giammo. Explain the therapeutic effects of atorvastatin.

20. What type of lifestyle modifications should the nurse discuss with Mrs. Giammo (and her husband) prior to discharge?

Mr. Aponi

GENDER

Male

AGE

85

SETTING

- Long-term care

ETHNICITY

- Native American

CULTURAL CONSIDERATIONS

- Touch; nonverbal behavior

PREEXISTING CONDITION

- Progressive dementia over the past seven years

COEXISTING CONDITION

- Urinary incontinence

COMMUNICATION

- Impaired communication secondary to altered mental status

DISABILITY

- Unable to care for himself independently due to cognitive decline

SOCIOECONOMIC

- Lives in a long-term care facility; wife passed away five years ago; he has no children

SPIRITUAL/RELIGIOUS

PHARMACOLOGIC

LEGAL

ETHICAL

ALTERNATIVE THERAPY

PRIORITIZATION

DELEGATION

EASY

THE NERVOUS/NEUROLOGICAL SYSTEM

Level of difficulty: Easy

Overview: This case requires the nurse to distinguish the difference between dementia and delirium and plan nursing care accordingly. How the client's cultural beliefs impact care is considered.

Client Profile

Mr. Aponi has a history of dementia. His dementia limits his ability to respond appropriately to questions and at times Mr. Aponi is easily agitated and resistant to nursing care. He refuses to take his medications, spitting them back out, gripping the bedside rail when the nurse tries to turn him, and yelling out for his wife to save him.

Case Study

Mr. Aponi is an 85-year-old man with a history of dementia. He is a resident of a long-term facility. Mr. Aponi's frequent incontinence necessitates the development of therapeutic communication to facilitate activities of daily living (ADL) care and frequent skin hygiene. The nurse caring for Mr. Aponi for the first time soon learns that talking slowly and softly is the most effective way of focusing the client's attention and prompting him to follow basic instructions such as turning side to side. The nurse feels uneasy about speaking to Mr. Aponi as if he were a child in some ways. However, the nurse finds that this manner of speech keeps Mr. Aponi calm and that he responds well to praise and compliments and that he is very helpful to the nurse in assisting with his own care.

On the second day of caring for him, the nurse notes that Mr. Aponi is more agitated and needs frequent reorientation regarding where he is. The nurse needs the assistance of another person to hold Mr. Aponi's arm steady while assessing his blood pressure since Mr. Aponi keeps pulling his arm away yelling "no." At one point in the day, Mr. Aponi tells the nurse, "There was a little boy in the room a minute ago. Where did he go?" The nurse knows there was not a little boy in the room, but does not know how to respond. The nurse ignores Mr. Aponi's comment and redirects his attention to what is on television.

When saying good-bye to Mr. Aponi at the end of the second day, the nurse is disappointed that Mr. Aponi does not seem to recognize the nurse or remember that the nurse has been caring for him for the past two days. The nurse is saddened to see him so confused and is emotionally exhausted after two days of responding to his frequent changes in behavior.

Questions

1. The nurse caring for Mr. Aponi overhears another nurse state, "Well, of course he is confused. He is 85 years old." How should Mr. Aponi's nurse respond?

2. Discuss the characteristics that define *delirium* and *dementia*. What is the principal difference between the diagnoses of delirium and dementia?

3. Describe the following strategies for caring for a confused client: validation, redirection, and reminiscence.

4. Explain why Mr. Aponi may state, "There was a little boy in the room a minute ago. Where did he go?" Which of the above strategies (in question 3) would be most effective in responding to his statement?

5. What are three nursing diagnoses appropriate for Mr. Aponi's plan of care?

6. Discuss the importance of nonverbal communication when communicating with a person who is confused and agitated. Consider Mr. Aponi's ethnicity.

Mrs. Greene

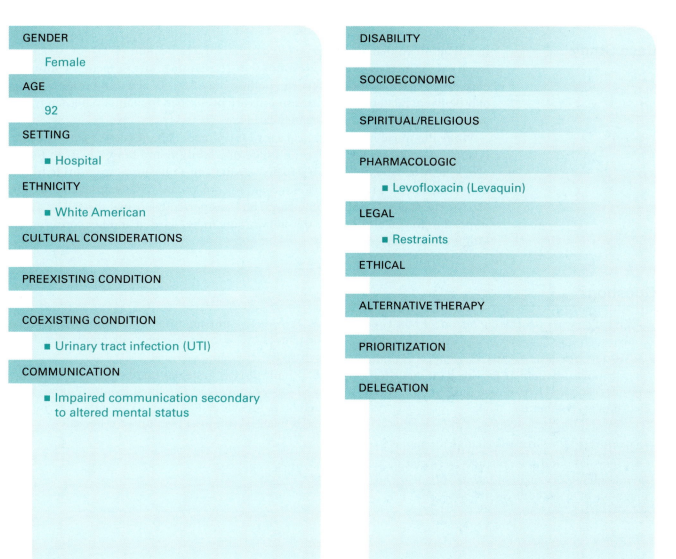

GENDER

Female

AGE

92

SETTING

- Hospital

ETHNICITY

- White American

CULTURAL CONSIDERATIONS

PREEXISTING CONDITION

COEXISTING CONDITION

- Urinary tract infection (UTI)

COMMUNICATION

- Impaired communication secondary to altered mental status

DISABILITY

SOCIOECONOMIC

SPIRITUAL/RELIGIOUS

PHARMACOLOGIC

- Levofloxacin (Levaquin)

LEGAL

- Restraints

ETHICAL

ALTERNATIVE THERAPY

PRIORITIZATION

DELEGATION

EASY

THE NERVOUS/NEUROLOGICAL SYSTEM

Level of difficulty: Easy

Overview: This case requires the nurse to recognize the most likely etiology of an acute change in mental status. Appropriate nursing interventions for a client requiring a physical restraint are considered.

Client Profile

Mrs. Greene is a 92-year-old woman who presents to the emergency room with an acute change in mental status and generalized weakness. Her past medical history is unremarkable. She has not had episodes of confusion in the past.

Case Study

It is determined that Mrs. Greene has a urinary tract infection (UTI) for which she is started on intravenous (IV) levofloxacin (Levaquin). Mrs. Greene's confusion escalates to visual hallucinations, the pulling out of two IV sites, and restless nights of little sleep. Bilateral soft wrist restraints are prescribed to maintain her safety, the integrity of the IV site, and the Foley catheter.

While the nurse is providing care for Mrs. Greene, Mrs. Greene's son visits. He is very distraught over Mrs. Greene's state of confusion and her inability to recognize him. Mrs. Greene is unable to answer her son's questions appropriately and frequently states, "I told you I do not want to cook today." Visibly upset and tearful, Mr. Greene states, "I don't understand. She was perfectly normal three days ago. I stopped by to visit and she was outside working in her garden and her conversation with me made perfect sense."

Questions

1. What do you suspect is the reason for Mrs. Greene's confusion?

2. Would you describe Mrs. Greene's confusion as delirium or dementia? Provide a rationale for your decision and explain the difference between delirium and dementia.

3. What are three appropriate nursing diagnoses that address Mrs. Greene's change in mental status?

4. State at least three outcome goals that should be included in the plan of care for Mrs. Greene's diagnosis of acute confusion.

5. Provide five nursing interventions to include in the plan of care for Mrs. Greene's diagnosis of acute confusion.

6. Briefly discuss strategies that help prevent the need for restraints. List five nursing interventions to include in Mrs. Greene's plan of care now that she needs bilateral soft wrist restraints for her safety.

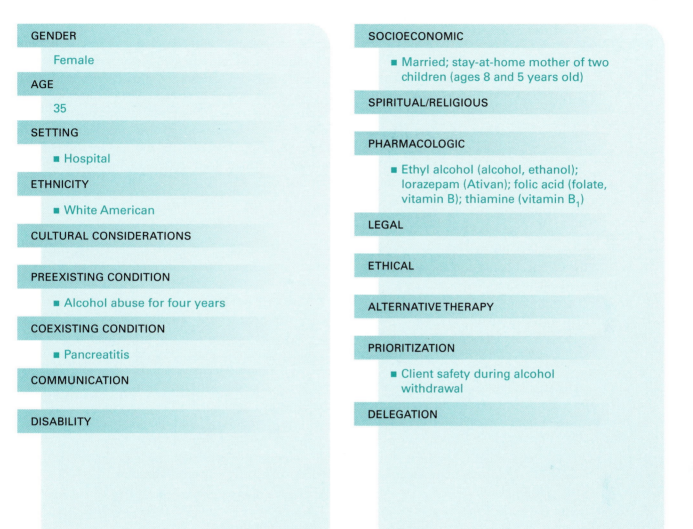

GENDER

Female

AGE

35

SETTING

■ Hospital

ETHNICITY

■ White American

CULTURAL CONSIDERATIONS

PREEXISTING CONDITION

■ Alcohol abuse for four years

COEXISTING CONDITION

■ Pancreatitis

COMMUNICATION

DISABILITY

SOCIOECONOMIC

■ Married; stay-at-home mother of two children (ages 8 and 5 years old)

SPIRITUAL/RELIGIOUS

PHARMACOLOGIC

■ Ethyl alcohol (alcohol, ethanol); lorazepam (Ativan); folic acid (folate, vitamin B); thiamine (vitamin B_1)

LEGAL

ETHICAL

ALTERNATIVE THERAPY

PRIORITIZATION

■ Client safety during alcohol withdrawal

DELEGATION

MODERATE

THE NERVOUS/NEUROLOGICAL SYSTEM

Level of difficulty: Moderate

Overview: The nurse in this case is asked to define terminology associated with alcohol abuse and discuss the effects alcohol has on the body. This case requires that the nurse recognize the initial manifestations of alcohol withdrawal and anticipate the symptoms the client may exhibit while hospitalized. The use of lorazepam (Ativan) and rationale for folic acid (folate, vitamin B) and thiamine (vitamin B_1) supplementation in the treatment of alcohol withdrawal is reviewed. The pertinent Healthy People 2010 health promotion considerations for the client are identified.

Client Profile

Mrs. Perry is a 35-year-old woman admitted to the hospital with pancreatitis. During her stay, Mrs. Perry experiences alcohol withdrawal.

Case Study

Mrs. Perry arrives at the emergency department with complaints of severe abdominal pain. She is admitted to the nursing unit at noon with a diagnosis of pancreatitis. While completing the nursing admission assessment, Mrs. Perry tells the day shift nurse that she drinks "a couple of cases of beer each week." She states her last drink was this morning. While doing rounds, the evening shift nurse notices that Mrs. Perry has tremors and is very anxious and restless. Her vital signs are blood pressure 130/82, pulse rate 88, respiratory rate 16, and temperature 99.6°F (37.5°C). The health care provider is notified. Daily folic acid and thiamine, and lorazepam as needed, are prescribed.

Questions

1. Briefly discuss the classification, metabolism, and excretion of alcohol.

2. Provide a definition for each of the following terms associated with alcohol use: *psychoactive substance, addiction, blackout, detoxification, intoxication, overdose, recidivism, sobriety, substance abuse, substance dependence, tolerance,* and *withdrawal.*

3. What are the characteristic effects of alcohol on the body?

4. What is considered the legal blood alcohol intoxication level in most of the United States?

5. Discuss the potential life-threatening complications associated with acute alcohol intoxication. What causes these complications?

6. When should the nurse expect the manifestations of alcohol withdrawal to begin and what symptoms will the nurse anticipate in the next few days?

7. What are delirium tremens (DTs)? Discuss the life-threatening complications of DTs.

8. Why is lorazepam (Ativan) prescribed as part of the management of Mrs. Perry's alcohol withdrawal? Discuss the most effective administration schedule of lorazepam (Ativan) for Mrs. Perry.

9. Provide a rationale for the prescription of folic acid (folate, vitamin B) and thiamine (vitamin B_1) in the management of alcohol withdrawal.

10. Generate five possible nursing diagnoses to address Mrs. Perry's alcohol withdrawal.

11. Discuss the Healthy People 2010 goal pertinent in Mrs. Perry's case and Mrs. Perry's health promotion priorities.

CASE STUDY 6

Mr. Cooper

GENDER

Male

AGE

73

SETTING

- Home

ETHNICITY

- White American

CULTURAL CONSIDERATIONS

PREEXISTING CONDITION

COEXISTING CONDITION

COMMUNICATION

- No answering machine; slurred speech

DISABILITY

- Progressive, degenerative disease

SOCIOECONOMIC

- Lives alone; non-smoker

SPIRITUAL/RELIGIOUS

PHARMACOLOGIC

- Ibuprofen (Motrin); riluzole (Rilutek)

LEGAL

- Advance directive

ETHICAL

ALTERNATIVE THERAPY

- Palliative care

PRIORITIZATION

- End-of-life planning

DELEGATION

- Collaboration between health care provider, home care nurse, home care physical therapist (PT), home care occupational therapist (OT), speech-language pathologist (SLP)

THE NERVOUS/NEUROLOGICAL SYSTEM

Level of difficulty: Difficult

Overview: This case explores the onset and diagnosis of ALS. Management of ALS with regard to medication and an interdisciplinary team approach is discussed. The nurse must consider how the prognosis of ALS will affect the client and his family. End-of-life issues are addressed.

Client Profile

Mr. Cooper is a 73-year-old man with no significant past medical history. He lives alone and is very independent in function and spirit. He was seen in the emergency department six weeks ago for complaints of "arthritis in his right knee." He was examined, given a prescription for ibuprofen, provided with a cane, and instructed to follow up with his health care provider. When Mr. Cooper sees his health care provider for his follow-up visit, the health care provider notices that as Mr. Cooper enters the examination room, he has right footdrop. When the health care provider asks Mr. Cooper what has brought him in today, Mr. Cooper states "I have arthritis in this right knee." Mr. Cooper explains that he has had this "arthritis" for three months. However, when asked about pain in the knee, Mr. Cooper denies any pain and states "well, maybe it's a nerve problem." On physical exam, his vital signs are within normal limits and consistent with Mr. Cooper's baseline. The health care provider notes that Mr. Cooper has no strength or power in his right lower extremity from the knee down. There is increased tone in his upper right extremity, indicating that those muscles are tighter than they should be. The health care provider also notices hyperreflexia. The health care provider prescribes a head computed tomography (CT) scan and multiple blood tests. The results of the CT scan and blood tests are all within normal limits. An urgent referral to a neurologist is made, and the health care provider asks the nurse to arrange for Mr. Cooper to have magnetic resonance imagery (MRI) of his head and neck and an electromyelogram (EMG). The nurse plans to arrange dates for these tests and to call Mr. Cooper with instructions. Mr. Cooper is fitted for an ankle-foot orthosis (AFO) brace and home physical therapy is arranged as prescribed by the health care provider.

Case Study

The nurse attempts to notify Mr. Cooper of the dates, times, and instructions regarding his MRI and EMG. However, Mr. Cooper does not have an answering machine. The health care provider is notified and she decides to call Mr. Cooper from home to see if she can reach him at home and give him the information. When the health care provider calls Mr. Cooper, he is speaking with slurred speech. The health care provider asks Mr. Cooper how long he has had difficulty speaking clearly to which Mr. Cooper replies, "I just have a touch of laryngitis is all." Mr. Cooper denies a cough, runny nose, fever, discomfort in his throat, and dysphagia. Concerned, the health care provider suggests that Mr. Cooper go to the emergency department for an evaluation. Despite the health care provider's repeated suggestions, Mr. Cooper refuses.

The next day, the health care provider calls Mr. Cooper's home physical therapist and asks the therapist to call her during the visit and let her know if Mr. Cooper is still exhibiting slurred speech. Later that morning, the physical therapist notifies the health care provider that indeed Mr. Cooper continues to have slurred speech. Per the health care provider's request, Mr. Cooper is transported to the emergency department. An MRI is unrevealing. However, an EMG is consistent with amyotrophic lateral sclerosis (ALS).

Questions

1. What is footdrop and why does it occur in a person with ALS?

2. An AFO brace is prescribed for Mr. Cooper. What does this brace do?

3. An EMG is prescribed for Mr. Cooper. Does this test require his consent? Explain this test to Mr. Cooper and provide instruction regarding anything he should do to prepare for this test.

4. Mr. Cooper, who is with his daughter, asks the nurse "What is ALS? Is it a type of arthritis like I thought?" It can be a sad and emotionally difficult explanation to give, but how would you explain the diagnosis to Mr. Cooper? Include in your discussion the symptoms, cause, incidence, and usual age of onset.

5. What is the prognosis for Mr. Cooper?

6. Riluzole is prescribed for Mr. Cooper. Explain how this medication works. What are the benefits of its use in clients with ALS?

7. Mr. Cooper is prescribed riluzole 50 mg PO every twelve hours. The nurse is teaching Mr. Cooper about his new medication. What should the nurse tell him about how to take riluzole with regard to timing and missed doses? Offer dietary suggestions to maximize the effects of riluzole.

8. Mr. Cooper lives alone but his daughter and family live close by. The nurse is pleased to learn that the daughter (and family) will be involved in Mr. Cooper's care and be a support system for him as he copes with his disease. Discuss the issues and arrangements the nurse should address with Mr. Cooper and his daughter, considering Mr. Cooper's prognosis.

9. Describe the purpose of the following advance directive alternatives: living will, health care proxy or durable power of attorney, and an advance care medical directive.

10. Discuss the concerns regarding Mr. Cooper's slurred speech. With whom should the nurse collaborate to help Mr. Cooper?

11. The nurse will collaborate with the home care physical therapist to develop an exercise and mobility program and ensure Mr. Cooper's safety in his home. Create a list of at least five components of a safe home environment.

12. An occupational therapist will work with Mr. Cooper to help him with strategies to maintain his independence with activities of daily living (ADLs) for as long as possible. Discuss at least five pieces of equipment available to assist Mr. Cooper with his ADLs.

13. Identify three nursing diagnoses appropriate for Mr. Cooper's plan of care following his diagnosis of ALS.

14. Identify three nursing diagnoses appropriate for Mr. Cooper's plan of care as his ALS progresses.

15. What is palliative care?

16. Why do you think Mr. Cooper self-diagnosed himself with "arthritis" and "laryngitis"?

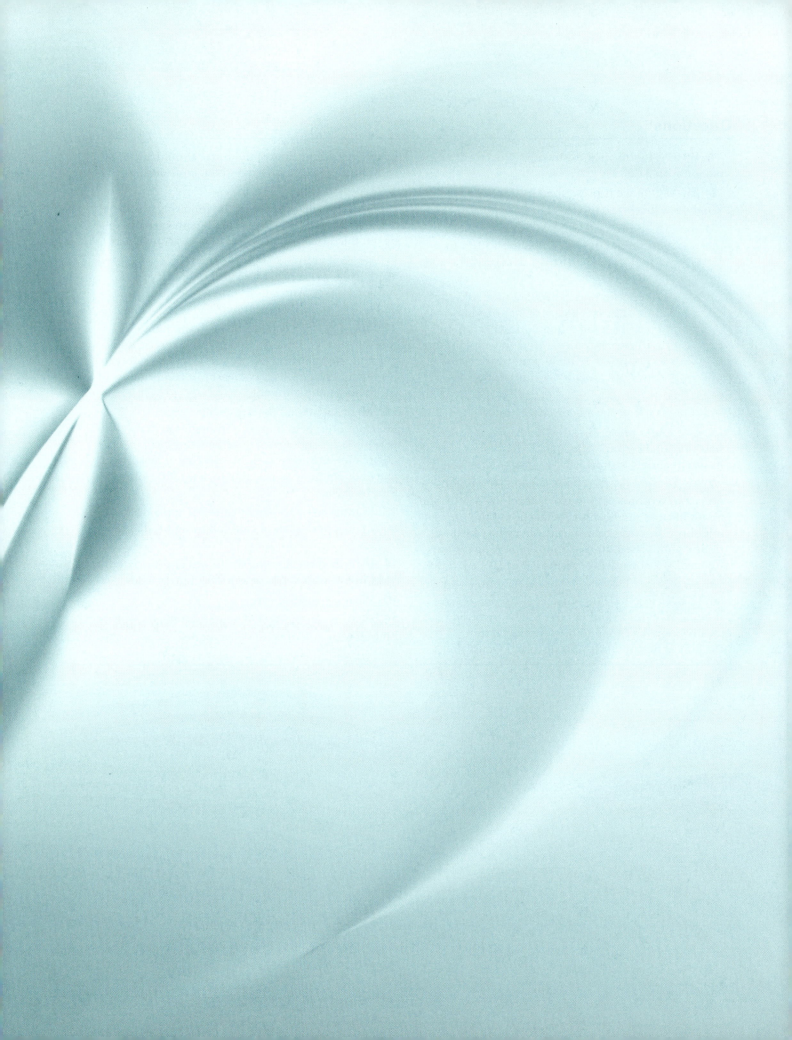

PART FOUR

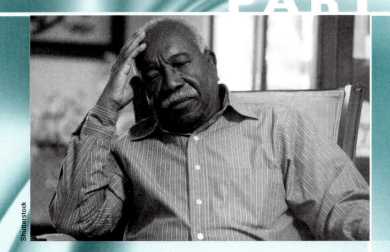

The Sensory System

Mr. Evans

GENDER

Male

AGE

73

SETTING

- Outpatient clinic

ETHNICITY

- Black American

CULTURAL CONSIDERATIONS

PREEXISTING CONDITIONS

- Diabetes mellitus type 2; hypertension

COEXISTING CONDITIONS

- Anxiety; depression

COMMUNICATION

DISABILITY

- Visual difficulties

SOCIOECONOMIC

- Recent death of wife

SPIRITUAL/RELIGIOUS

PHARMACOLOGIC

- Zoloft; Glucophage; Hydrochlorothiazide

LEGAL

ETHICAL

ALTERNATIVE THERAPY

PRIORITIZATION

DELEGATION

MODERATE

THE SENSORY SYSTEM

Level of difficulty: Moderate

Overview: This case requires the nurse to discuss glaucoma symptoms, differentiating between primary and acute. An understanding of pharmacological treatments and surgical interventions is required. Nursing diagnoses for priority care are identified.

Client Profile

Mr. Evans is a 73-year-old man who presents to the clinic with complaints of "foggy" vision, headaches, and aching in his eyes. He also reports seeing "rings around lights." Since his wife's death two months ago, he states things have not been going well at home. He has not been able to handle the bill payments because of his change in vision and his depression. He is upset and is worried that he will not be able to stay in his home. His children live in another state and have not been home to help him.

Case Study

Mr. Evans's vital signs are temperature 98.1°F, blood pressure 172/92, pulse 68, and respiratory rate of 24. Tonometry shows an elevated intraocular pressure of 26 mm Hg. He reports that his peripheral vision is decreased and it is noted in the visual exam by the physician that his optic disk appears pale and the depth and size of the optic cup appears increased. Mr. Evans's history reveals that his mother also had glaucoma. His neighbor and good friend is with him and states, "I take care of Mr. Evans and drive for him." His diabetes is under control and he states, "If I keep good track of my diet and blood sugars, the only medication I need is my morning diabetic pill." He also talks openly about how depressed he has been since his wife died.

Questions

1. Define glaucoma and the group of conditions that can cause it.

2. Describe the tonometry test and normal results. What other tests can be used in diagnostics?

3. What symptoms would be found with acute angle-closure glaucoma?

4. The medical diagnosis for Mr. Evans is primary open-angle glaucoma. What are the clues in the case study that support this diagnosis?

5. What risk factors does Mr. Evans have that contribute to glaucoma?

6. Discuss the pharmaceutical management for glaucoma. Discuss teaching Mr. Evans about these medications.

7. Mr. Evans has surgical management with a laser trabeculoplasty after failure of nonsurgical management. What is laser trabeculoplasty? What would be further management if he failed to respond to the laser therapy?

8. List three priority nursing diagnoses for Mr. Evans.

9. Mr. Evans has many worries about his ability to manage at home. What are main primary nursing foci for an older adult with impaired vision? What types of services would help him to remain in his own home?

PART FIVE

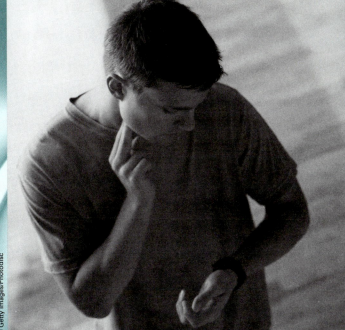

The Integumentary System

Mrs. Sweeney

GENDER

Female

AGE

70

SETTING

- Home

ETHNICITY

- White American

CULTURAL CONSIDERATIONS

PREEXISTING CONDITION

- Stroke ten months ago with right-sided weakness

COEXISTING CONDITIONS

- Urinary incontinence; impaired mobility

COMMUNICATION

DISABILITY

- Right-sided weakness; ambulates with a walker

SOCIOECONOMIC

- Lives alone in a first-floor apartment

SPIRITUAL/RELIGIOUS

PHARMACOLOGIC

LEGAL

ETHICAL

ALTERNATIVE THERAPY

PRIORITIZATION

- Educating client and caregiver to promote skin integrity

DELEGATION

THE INTEGUMENTARY SYSTEM

Level of difficulty: Easy

Overview: This case requires that the nurse understand the impact of incontinence on impaired skin integrity. The nurse teaches the client and primary caregiver ways to minimize episodes of incontinence and promote good skin care.

Client Profile   **Mrs. Sweeney** is a 70-year-old woman who had a stroke less than a year ago. Mrs. Sweeney is alert and oriented. She feels the sensation to void, but right-sided weakness prevents her from always being able to get to the bathroom in time. For this reason, she wears incontinence undergarments. Mrs. Sweeney's daughter, Adele, stops by twice each day to check on Mrs. Sweeney and prepare meals for her. There are times when Mrs. Sweeney is incontinent and remains in a wet undergarment until Adele comes to visit.

Case Study   While assisting Mrs. Sweeney in the bathroom, Adele notices that Mrs. Sweeney's coccyx and perineum area are reddened and excoriated. Adele learns that Mrs. Sweeney sometimes sits in a wet undergarment until she arrives. Mrs. Sweeney explains, "I know I am wet. It is just easier to wait for you to get here than to try and change the undergarment myself." Adele is concerned. She calls a local visiting nurses association to get some information about how to manage Mrs. Sweeney's incontinence and asks if there is any skin therapy to reduce the redness.

Questions

1. Describe at least three factors that affect voiding and may result in incontinence in an adult.

2. What is incontinence? Describe the characteristics of each of the six types of urinary incontinence: *stress, reflex, urge, functional, total* (chronic incontinence), and *transient* (acute incontinence).

3. Which type of incontinence does Mrs. Sweeney have and what data support the diagnosis?

4. Mrs. Sweeney tells the nurse, "I try to limit the amount of fluid I drink to one or two small glasses a day so that I do not have to go to the bathroom as much." What teaching should the nurse provide in response to Mrs. Sweeney's comment?

5. Explain at least three factors that are contributing to Mrs. Sweeney's impaired skin integrity.

6. What will the visiting nurse most likely tell Mrs. Sweeney and Adele to consider in an effort to minimize Mrs. Sweeney's incontinent episodes?

7. What are three suggestions the visiting nurse will include while teaching Adele to care for Mrs. Sweeney's skin?

8. List five nursing diagnoses that are appropriate for Mrs. Sweeney.

CASE STUDY 2

Mr. Dennis

EASY

GENDER

Male

AGE

57

SETTING

- Hospital

ETHNICITY

- White American

CULTURAL CONSIDERATIONS

PREEXISTING CONDITION

COEXISTING CONDITION

- Herpes zoster infection

COMMUNICATION

DISABILITY

SOCIOECONOMIC

SPIRITUAL/RELIGIOUS

PHARMACOLOGIC

- Oxycodone/acetaminophen (Percocet); acyclovir (Zovirax); hydrocortisone (Sarna HC); famciclovir (Famvir); valacyclovir hydrochloride (Valtrex); gabapentin (Neurontin); triamcinolone (Aristocort, Kenacort, Kenalog); aluminum sulfate (Domeboro)

LEGAL

ETHICAL

ALTERNATIVE THERAPY

- Cutaneous stimulation; distraction

PRIORITIZATION

- Pain management

DELEGATION

- Client assignment considerations to avoid client care by pregnant staff members

THE INTEGUMENTARY SYSTEM

Level of difficulty: Easy

Overview: Although in pain, the client refuses medication for fear of becoming addicted. The nurse provides teaching to clarify the myths and facts of pain medication and provide alternatives to pharmacological pain management. Treatment options for herpes zoster are discussed. Client assignments are considered to reduce the risks of exposure for pregnant staff.

63

Client Profile

Mr. Dennis is a 57-year-old man admitted with pain secondary to herpes zoster. He describes the pain as "agonizing" and states, "I feel like my skin is burning." The health care provider has prescribed acyclovir (Zovirax) and oxycodone/acetaminophen (Percocet) for Mr. Dennis. Mr. Dennis is reluctant to ask for the pain medication. He states, "I do not even want to start with that stuff. I have heard you can become addicted to pain medication very easily."

Case Study

The nurse sits with Mr. Dennis and discusses with him the common myths surrounding pain management and pain medications. Education regarding nonpharmacologic pain management strategies results in instruction on how to use distraction. The nurse also brings Mr. Dennis a cooling pad to facilitate pain management through cutaneous stimulation. Mr. Dennis feels better now about asking for his prescribed pain medication. Now that he is receiving (oxycodone/acetaminophen) Percocet on a regular basis in conjunction with alternative pain management strategies, he states his pain "has decreased considerably."

Questions

1. What is herpes zoster? Briefly discuss its cause and incidence.

2. Discuss the characteristic manifestations of herpes zoster and its typical progression and healing time. What would a diagnosis of "ophthalmic herpes zoster" indicate?

3. Mr. Dennis describes his initial pain as "agonizing" and then states his pain has decreased "considerably." Discuss the assessment tools that help quantify the subjective experience of pain.

4. Create two columns. In the first column, provide at least three myths about the pain experience and the use of pain medication. In the second column, provide a fact that dispels each myth.

5. Discuss how the nurse can facilitate effective pain management for Mr. Dennis.

6. Describe cutaneous stimulation as an alternative pain management strategy.

7. Describe the use of distraction as an alternative pain management strategy.

8. Discuss the focus of treatment and treatment options for herpes zoster. Consider acute treatment, as well as long-term treatment of postherpetic neuralgia.

9. Help the nurse generate two appropriate nursing diagnoses for Mr. Dennis's plan of care.

10. When creating the client assignment, the charge nurse purposely does not assign Mr. Dennis to a pregnant staff nurse. Discuss the potential risks associated with a pregnant woman's exposure to herpes zoster, and the method and time frame during which the infected client can transmit the virus to others.

GENDER

Female

AGE

72

SETTING

- Hospital

ETHNICITY

- White American

CULTURAL CONSIDERATIONS

PREEXISTING CONDITIONS

- Heart failure (HF); stroke with subsequent right-sided hemiplegia

COEXISTING CONDITIONS

- MRSA (methicillin-resistant *Staphylococcus aureus*); receiving nutrition via a g-tube

COMMUNICATION

DISABILITY

- Needs complete assistance with ADLs and turning and repositioning

SOCIOECONOMIC

- Cost containment to decrease financial burden on health care system

SPIRITUAL/RELIGIOUS

PHARMACOLOGIC

- Mupirocin (Bactroban); vancomycin (Vancocin)

LEGAL

- OSHA guidelines

ETHICAL

- Noncompliance with contact precaution policies

ALTERNATIVE THERAPY

PRIORITIZATION

- Nursing organization and time management

DELEGATION

- Delegating retrieval of equipment and supplies

MODERATE

THE INTEGUMENTARY SYSTEM

Level of difficulty: Moderate

Overview: This case requires that the student nurse understand the transmission of nosocomial infections and initiate appropriate isolation precautions for MRSA. Treatment options for MRSA are explored. The student nurse serves as a client advocate by recognizing the importance of compliance with proper contact precautions by visitors and health care personnel. The importance of developing good time management and delegation skills is discussed. Finally, the financial burden of caring for a client with MRSA is considered with regard to the nurse's responsibility for cost containment.

Client Profile

Mrs. Sims is a 72-year-old female admitted with heart failure. Her heart failure has been resolved. Mrs. Sims needs complete care with her activities of daily living (ADLs) and with repositioning. Arrangements were being made for her discharge back to the long-term care facility when lab results revealed she is positive for MRSA in her urine. Mrs. Sims is in a private room and has been placed on contact precautions. Vancomycin is prescribed with peak and trough labs.

Case Study

The student nurse caring for Mrs. Sims follows the contact precaution guidelines as indicated by a sign outside of Mrs. Sims's door. The student nurse dons the personal protective equipment (PPE) located in a precaution cart outside the room. Once in the room to take a set of morning vital signs, the student nurse notices that there is not a separate blood pressure cuff or stethoscope assigned to the client. The student nurse removes the PPE and finds the staff nurse assigned to the client to ask for a blood pressure cuff and stethoscope. The staff nurse is able to locate a disposable stethoscope to remain in the client's room, but not a blood pressure cuff. The staff nurse instructs the student to use the unit's electronic blood pressure machine and to wash it thoroughly with antibacterial wipes after each use.

Throughout the day, the student realizes how much additional time is necessary to complete each care need for Mrs. Sims because, before entering the room, the student must don the PPE. The student also makes note of several precaution carts lining the hallway and realizes how prevalent infectious diseases are on this one hospital unit alone.

The student is pleased to see that when family members come to visit, they take the time to put on the proper PPE and remind new visitors to do the same. However, the student nurse notices that other nursing staff, housekeeping personnel, and the health care provider enter the room on several occasions without putting on the required equipment.

Questions

1. What is MRSA?

2. How is MRSA transmitted?

3. What are five nursing interventions that will help minimize the spread of MRSA while caring for Mrs. Sims?

4. Was it appropriate for the staff nurse to instruct the student nurse to use the unit's electronic blood pressure machine and wash it thoroughly with antibacterial wipes after each use? Explain why or why not.

5. Discuss the importance of efficiency in gathering needed supplies and time management when caring for a client on contact precautions.

6. Discuss appropriate delegation to others when the student nurse requires additional supplies or equipment once in the client's room.

7. What treatment options are there to help resolve Mrs. Sims's MRSA?

8. Mrs. Sims is taking vancomycin (Vancocin). A peak and trough is ordered. Explain peak and trough levels and the purpose of these laboratory tests.

9. What diagnostic test(s) will be done to confirm negative or positive MRSA infection prior to Mrs. Sims's discharge to the long-term care facility?

10. Discuss the ethical considerations for hospital personnel regarding compliance with contact precautions?

11. What could the nursing student do to help facilitate greater compliance with the contact precautions by staff caring for and entering Mrs. Sims's room?

12. Discuss the financial considerations of caring for a client with MRSA.

13. List two nursing diagnoses appropriate for the plan of care for a client with MRSA.

CASE STUDY 4

Mr. Vincent

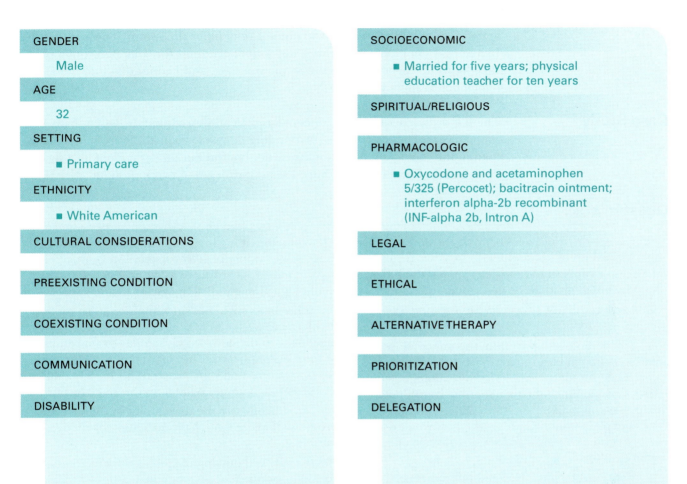

GENDER

Male

AGE

32

SETTING

- Primary care

ETHNICITY

- White American

CULTURAL CONSIDERATIONS

PREEXISTING CONDITION

COEXISTING CONDITION

COMMUNICATION

DISABILITY

SOCIOECONOMIC

- Married for five years; physical education teacher for ten years

SPIRITUAL/RELIGIOUS

PHARMACOLOGIC

- Oxycodone and acetaminophen 5/325 (Percocet); bacitracin ointment; interferon alpha-2b recombinant (INF-alpha 2b, Intron A)

LEGAL

ETHICAL

ALTERNATIVE THERAPY

PRIORITIZATION

DELEGATION

THE INTEGUMENTARY SYSTEM

Level of difficulty: Difficult

Overview: This case requires the nurse to recognize the risk factors and characteristics of melanoma. The diagnostic process and treatment options for a malignant skin lesion are discussed. The nurse considers the client's need for emotional support.

Client Profile

Mr. Vincent is a 32-year-old man who has scheduled an appointment with a dermatologist to have a black spot on his right ear assessed. Mr. Vincent states, "My wife noticed a black circular area on my ear about two weeks ago and she suggested I get it looked at since she did not remember the spot being there before. I know that too much time in the sun is not very good for your skin. I'm a physical education teacher so I am out in the sun a lot, and I admit that I do not always remember to apply sunscreen."

Case Study

There is a dark area on Mr. Vincent's right ear approximately 0.4 cm by 0.4 cm round in size. The color of the surrounding skin is normal. Mr. Vincent says that he noticed the spot about four months earlier but did not think much of it. "I figured it was a mole. Since it did not hurt, I really didn't give it much thought."

Questions

1. You are the nurse working with the dermatologist. Make a list of questions you could ask regarding the area of concern to help determine if the site on Mr. Vincent's ear could be melanoma.

2. Explain the ABCD criteria for assessing a skin lesion.

3. The pathology report from the punch biopsy states, "deep penetrating nevi with atypical features worrisome for melanoma." The dermatologist suggests that Mr. Vincent have a sentinel lymph node mapping and biopsy procedure. How might the nurse explain what this procedure is, why it is done, and potential common and serious adverse effects/complications?

4. Mrs. Vincent says, "How did this happen? My husband has dark hair and olive skin. I thought only fair-skinned redheads got skin cancer." Is there any truth to Mrs. Vincent's assumption? List five risk factors the nurse should include in an explanation of what puts individuals at greater risk for skin cancer.

5. Discuss the incidence of dark-skinned individuals diagnosed with melanoma.

6. The results of the sentinel lymph node mapping and biopsy reveal that the most proximal lymph node near Mr. Vincent's parotid gland is positive with a 0.1 mm micrometastasis. Given that the punch biopsy was suspicious for melanoma and that there is a positive sentinel lymph node, the dermatologist prescribes a CT scan of the head, chest, neck, abdomen, thorax, and pelvis, a MRI of the brain, and a PET scan of the body to determine the extent of Mr. Vincent's melanoma. Mr. Vincent asks, "What gland is it near?" and then states, "I know what a CT scan and MRI are but what is a PET scan?" What function does the parotid gland serve? Explain a PET scan to Mr. Vincent.

7. What does it mean to explain cancer according to its "stage" using the TNM system? Melanoma may be staged according to a "clinical stage" and a "pathological stage." Briefly discuss the difference.

8. It has been six weeks since his initial visit to the dermatologist and Mr. and Mrs. Vincent are meeting with the dermatologist today to get results of the diagnostic tests. They learn that Mr. Vincent has been diagnosed with "Stage IIIA T1a, N1a, M0" malignant melanoma. What does this stage mean?

9. Mr. Vincent asks the dermatologist, "What is my prognosis?" What is Mr. Vincent's five-year survival rate?

10. Identify two nursing diagnoses the nurse should consider for Mr. Vincent when he learns of his diagnosis of melanoma.

11. Discuss what the nurse can do to reduce the fear and anxiety that Mr. Vincent may feel upon learning that he has melanoma.

12. Results of Mr. Vincent's CT scan, MRI, and PET scan are negative. The suggested intervention is a curative lymph node dissection. There are no postoperative complications and Mr. Vincent is being discharged home. He is given a prescription for oxycodone and acetaminophen 5/325 one to two tablets every four to six hours as needed for postsurgical incisional pain. He has staples at his incision site to which Bacitracin is applied and the site is covered with a sterile dressing. He will return to the surgeon's office two days after discharge to have the dressing removed and a postoperative incision check. The nurse is providing discharge teaching. What are the common adverse effects of oxycodone and acetaminophen 5/325 and instructions for safe administration? What warning signs indicate that Mr. Vincent should call his surgeon?

Questions (continued)

13. Identify two nursing diagnoses the nurse should consider for Mr. Vincent following his lymph node dissection.

14. Four weeks later, Mr. Vincent sees an oncologist to discuss recommendations regarding adjunct treatment. The oncologist explains that the only FDA-approved therapy for stage III melanoma is high-dose interferon (INF)-alpha 2b, which offers a modest survival benefit with the risk of adverse effects. What are the adverse effects of high-dose interferon (INF)-alpha 2b?

15. The oncologist suggests Mr. Vincent also consider treatment offered through participation in a clinical trial. What is a clinical trial and what are the three phases of a clinical trial?

16. Mr. Vincent does some research and takes some time to consider the treatment options and discuss them with his wife. He decides that presented with only the possibility, and not a guarantee, of an increase in survival rate with the interferon therapy, the benefit does not outweigh the risk of the adverse effects. He declines interferon treatment and is going to explore clinical trials. As Mr. Vincent's nurse, how should you respond to Mr. Vincent's decision?

17. What will Mr. Vincent require in terms of follow-up care? Discuss how often Mr. Vincent will need to see the dermatologist, the symptoms to report, precautions to take, and the need for emotional support.

Mr. Lee

GENDER

Male

AGE

55

SETTING

- Hospital

ETHNICITY

- Black American

CULTURAL CONSIDERATIONS

PREEXISTING CONDITION

- Head trauma three months ago

COEXISTING CONDITION

- Recent seizure

COMMUNICATION

DISABILITY

- Potential long-term complications

SOCIOECONOMIC

SPIRITUAL/RELIGIOUS

PHARMACOLOGIC

- Phenytoin (Dilantin)

LEGAL

ETHICAL

ALTERNATIVE THERAPY

PRIORITIZATION

- Adverse medication reaction

DELEGATION

THE INTEGUMENTARY SYSTEM

Level of difficulty: Difficult

Overview: This case requires the nurse to implement strategies to maintain the client's safety in the event of a seizure. The nurse also must recognize the signs and symptoms of an adverse reaction to a medication. The client must be transferred to the appropriate level of care. Treatment goals and priority nursing diagnoses are reviewed.

DIFFICULT

Client Profile   **Mr. Lee** is a 55-year-old man with a history of head trauma three months ago after falling from a ladder. He is seen in the emergency department today after experiencing a seizure at work. Mr. Lee received a loading dose of phenytoin in the emergency department and is admitted for a thorough work-up.

Case Study   Upon arrival to the nursing unit, Mr. Lee is alert and oriented but lethargic. The following day, Mr. Lee has received two doses of phenytoin, and he has not had a seizure since admission. His lethargy has resolved. Midafternoon, Mr. Lee calls for the nurse. He shows the nurse his arms and hands and asks, "Look at these red splotches and blisters. What do you think this is from?" The nurse asks Mr. Lee if he has any other symptoms. He replies, "My eyes are itchy and burning and my throat is a little sore. Maybe I am allergic to the laundry detergent the hospital uses to wash the bed sheets." Assessment reveals symmetric reddish-purple macules and bullae on his arms, hands, chest, and back. Mr. Lee's vital signs are within normal limits except his temperature, which is 102.1°F (38.9°C).

Questions

1. Should the nurse be concerned that upon arrival to the nursing unit Mr. Lee is lethargic?

2. What is the rationale for prescribing phenytoin for Mr. Lee?

3. Mr. Lee's plan of care includes seizure precautions. Explain how the nurse implements these precautions.

4. What do you believe is the cause of Mr. Lee's skin condition?

5. Discuss three critical interventions upon diagnosing Mr. Lee's reaction.

6. Mr. Lee is transferred to the burn unit. Explain the rationale for this transfer.

7. Identify four treatment goals the nurse will include while documenting Mr. Lee's plan of care.

8. Mr. Lee's wife notices that the nurse checked the thermostat in Mr. Lee's room even though Mr. Lee did not express discomfort with the room temperature. Why was the nurse checking the temperature in the room?

9. Mr. Lee's laboratory results are hemoglobin (Hgb) 18 g/dL, hematocrit (Hct) 57%, potassium (K^+) 6.5 mEq/L; his sodium (Na^{2+}) level is 126 mEq/L; and his bicarbonate (HCO_3^-) is 15 mEq/L. Are these results within normal limits? If not, explain what is causing any abnormal result.

10. The nurse dons a protective gown, mask, gloves, and cap prior to changing Mr. Lee's dressings. Why is this precaution necessary?

11. Is Stevens Johnson Syndrome self-limiting or life threatening? Explain your answer.

12. Briefly discuss three potential complications the nurse will watch for as Stevens Johnson Syndrome progresses.

13. Mr. Lee's coworker comes to visit and brings a beautiful vase full of flowers from her garden. The nurse asks that the visitor not bring the floral arrangement into Mr. Lee's room. What is the rationale for the nurse's request?

14. Clients with Stevens Johnson Syndrome sometimes suffer long-term effects. Briefly discuss three long-term complications that may result.

15. Identify five nursing diagnoses appropriate for Mr. Lee's plan of care while being cared for on the burn unit. Prioritize the diagnoses you have identified.

16. While providing discharge teaching, what should the nurse tell Mr. Lee (and his family) about preventing a recurrence of this adverse medication reaction in the future?

17. What resource can the nurse suggest to help provide support once Mr. Lee is discharged from the hospital?

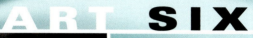

PART SIX

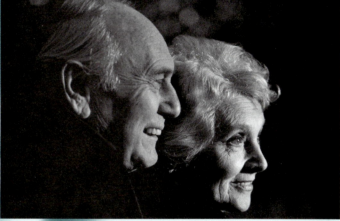

The Digestive System

GENDER

Female

AGE

46

SETTING

■ Hospital

ETHNICITY

■ White American

CULTURAL CONSIDERATIONS

PREEXISTING CONDITION

COEXISTING CONDITION

■ Urinary tract infection (UTI)

COMMUNICATION

DISABILITY

SOCIOECONOMIC

■ Married; no children

SPIRITUAL/RELIGIOUS

PHARMACOLOGIC

■ Cefoxitin sodium (Mefoxin); metronidazole (Flagyl); morphine sulfate; diphenoxylate hydrochloride with atropine sulfate (Lomotil); propantheline bromide (Pro-Banthine); acetaminophen (Tylenol)

LEGAL

ETHICAL

ALTERNATIVE THERAPY

PRIORITIZATION

DELEGATION

MODERATE

THE DIGESTIVE SYSTEM

Level of difficulty: Moderate

Overview: This case requires the nurse to recognize the clinical presentation of diverticular disease. The nurse is asked to compare the presenting symptoms of other differential diagnoses to those of diverticulitis. Diagnostic testing and the treatment of diverticulitis are discussed.

Client Profile   **Mrs. Dolan** is a 46-year-old female who presented to the emergency department with complaints of episodic abdominal pain, a low-grade fever, and diarrhea for almost two weeks. Mrs. Dolan was on vacation in another country when she developed pain in the left lower quadrant of her abdomen. Mrs. Dolan delayed seeking health care because of fear of the country's unfamiliar medical system and the assumption that bad water or food she had while on vacation must have given her a stomach "bug." Mrs. Dolan also reports a recent onset of painful urination.

Case Study   Upon examination in the emergency room, Mrs. Dolan is found to be dehydrated with a fever of 102.5°F (39.2 °C). Vital signs are blood pressure (BP) 106/58, pulse 88, and respiratory rate of 22. Her potassium (K^+) level is 2.8 mEq/L, erythrocyte sedimentation rate (ESR) is 37 mm/hr, and white blood cell (WBC) count is 16,000 cells/mm^3. A urinalysis showed a positive urinary tract infection (UTI) and an abdominal/pelvic computed tomography (CT) scan revealed diverticulitis with a question of an ileus.

Mrs. Dolan is admitted and started on intravenous (IV) fluid of D51/2 normal saline (NS) with 20 mEq of potassium chloride (KCl) at 50 mL per hour. Two IV antibiotics (cefoxitin sodium and metronidazole) are prescribed. Her admitting orders include nothing by mouth (NPO), bed rest, IV morphine sulfate for pain management, stools to be checked for occult blood, strict intake and output (I & O), and repeat blood work in the morning to monitor her K^+. Her height and weight on admission are 5 feet 7 inches and 170 lbs (77.3 kg). She is prescribed diphenoxylate hydrochloride with atropine sulfate, propantheline bromide, and acetaminophen as "as needed" pro re nata (prn) medications.

Questions

1. How does diverticulitis differ from diverticulosis?

2. Summarize the pathophysiology of acute and chronic diverticulitis.

3. Describe the predisposing risk factors for diverticulitis. Identify any contributing factors for the development of diverticulitis in Mrs. Dolan's case.

4. The emergency department health care provider also considered that Mrs. Dolan's symptoms could be indicative of a diagnosis of gastroenteritis. Briefly describe the clinical features of gastroenteritis and diverticulitis. How are the clinical presentations of these diagnoses similar?

5. What is the usual source of the bacteria that leads to the development of gastroenteritis?

6. Explain how Mrs. Dolan's symptoms might be related to her urinary tract infection.

7. The emergency department health care provider considered several differential diagnoses for Mrs. Dolan and a diagnosis of diverticulitis was determined. What diagnostic test confirmed Mrs. Dolan's diagnosis of acute diverticulitis?

8. Mrs. Dolan's abdominal/pelvic CT scan revealed diverticulitis with a question of an ileus. What is an ileus?

9. Briefly explain why a barium enema, sigmoidoscopy, and colonoscopy are not considered appropriate diagnostic tests for a client with suspected acute diverticulitis.

10. Discuss the medical management for a client with acute diverticulitis.

11. The admitting health care provider explains to Mr. and Mrs. Dolan that some clients require surgery if conservative treatment does not resolve the acute episode of diverticulitis. What are the indications for surgical intervention?

12. Discuss the rationale for including prn orders for diphenoxylate hydrochloride with atropine sulfate, propantheline bromide, and acetaminophen in Mrs. Dolan's treatment plan.

13. When collaborating with Mrs. Dolan to develop a plan of care, what outcome goals will be nursing care priorities?

14. Mrs. Dolan requests morphine sulfate. What should the nurse do before administering the medication?

Mrs. Dolan (Part 2)

GENDER

Female

AGE

46

SETTING

- Hospital

ETHNICITY

- White American

CULTURAL CONSIDERATIONS

PREEXISTING CONDITION

COEXISTING CONDITIONS

- Acute diverticulitis; urinary tract infection (UTI)

COMMUNICATION

DISABILITY

SOCIOECONOMIC

- Married; no children

SPIRITUAL/RELIGIOUS

- Catholic

PHARMACOLOGIC

- Nystatin (Mycostatin)

LEGAL

- Advance directive

ETHICAL

ALTERNATIVE THERAPY

PRIORITIZATION

- Emotional support; client education

DELEGATION

- Community resources

THE DIGESTIVE SYSTEM

Level of difficulty: Easy

Overview: This case requires the nurse to prepare Mr. and Mrs. Dolan for Mrs. Dolan's emergent surgical procedure. Following surgery, the nurse must provide discharge teaching to educate Mrs. Dolan on the care of her temporary colostomy. Priority nursing considerations for the client living with a colostomy are reviewed.

Client Profile

Mrs. Dolan is a 46-year-old female who presented to the emergency department three days ago with complaints of abdominal pain, fever, and diarrhea for almost two weeks. Upon examination in the emergency room, Mrs. Dolan was found to be dehydrated with a potassium (K^+) level of 2.8 mEq/L, erythrocyte sedimentation rate (ESR) of 37 mm/hr, and white blood cell (WBC) count of 16,000 cells/mm^3. She was positive for a urinary tract infection and an abdominal/pelvic computed tomography (CT) scan confirmed the diagnosis of diverticulitis. Mrs. Dolan was admitted to the hospital. She was started on intravenous (IV) fluids with potassium chloride (KCl) supplementation. She was also prescribed IV antibiotics and morphine sulfate for pain management. She has been nothing by mouth (NPO) since admission three days ago.

Case Study

After three days of IV fluids, antibiotics, and bowel rest, Mrs. Dolan's K^+ level is 3.7 mEq/L, ESR is 30 mm/hr, and WBC count is 15,000 cells/mm^3. Her vital signs are blood pressure (BP) 114/68, radial pulse/heart rate (HR) 102, respiratory rate (RR) 18, and temperature of 103°F (39.4°C). Mrs. Dolan has a follow-up abdominal/pelvic CT scan. The CT scan reveals that Mrs. Dolan's diverticultitis has not responded to conservative medical management and an abscess has developed. Surgical intervention is necessary and she is scheduled for surgery the next morning.

Questions

1. Briefly discuss the potential complications associated with acute diverticulitis.

2. Which assessment findings are of concern in Mrs. Dolan's case?

3. Describe Mrs. Dolan's preoperative care needs.

4. What are the potential complications associated with abdominal surgery that Mrs. Dolan should be informed of prior to giving consent for the surgical procedure?

5. Describe the purpose of the following advance directive alternatives: *living will, health care proxy* or *durable power of attorney,* and an *advance care medical directive.*

6. During the immediate postoperative phase of Mrs. Dolan's care, what should the nurse assess?

7. What is a *stoma* and how are the following three types of stomas surgically created: *end stoma, double-barrel stoma,* and *loop stoma?*

8. Generate two to three key points to address when providing Mrs. Dolan with colostomy care education regarding each of the following: *stoma assessment, skin protection, pouch care, diet, medications, sexuality issues,* and *community resources.*

9. Prioritize three nursing diagnoses appropriate for the client living with a colostomy.

CASE STUDY 3

Ms. Winnie

GENDER	**SPIRITUAL/RELIGIOUS**
Female	■ Jehovah's Witness
AGE	**PHARMACOLOGIC**
33	■ Norgestimate/ethinyl estradiol (Ortho Tri-Cyclen); ibuprofen (Advil); pantoprazole (Protonix); prochlorperazine (Compazine); omeprazole (Prilosec)
SETTING	
■ Hospital	
ETHNICITY	**LEGAL**
■ White American	
CULTURAL CONSIDERATIONS	**ETHICAL**
PREEXISTING CONDITION	**ALTERNATIVE THERAPY**
COEXISTING CONDITION	**PRIORITIZATION**
■ Flulike symptoms for one week	
COMMUNICATION	**DELEGATION**
	■ Delegating within the scope of assistant nursing personnel responsibilities
DISABILITY	
SOCIOECONOMIC	
■ Recently promoted to project manager	

THE DIGESTIVE SYSTEM

Level of difficulty: Moderate

Overview: This case requires recognition of the signs and symptoms of a gastrointestinal (GI) bleed and characteristics of upper versus lower GI tract bleeding. The nurse provides client education in preparation for a diagnostic procedure and explains the significance of the results. The procedure for administering a blood transfusion is reviewed. Discharge instructions are given.

Client Profile

Ms. Winnie is a 33-year-old woman who presented to the emergency department. She states, "I have been so sick. It must be the flu. Everyone at work has it. I am achy and tired. I keep vomiting and have not been able to keep anything down for the past three days. After a while, it is just these violent dry heaves since there is nothing more in my stomach to throw up. Tonight I vomited twice within three hours and it was red like blood. I got scared and came in."

Case Study

Ms. Winnie's vital signs are BP 110/60, HR 88, RR 20, temperature 100.5°F (38°C). Her skin is clammy and pale. Lab results are WBC 11,800 cells/mm^3, RBC 3.31 million/μL, Hgb 11 g/dL, Hct 34%, platelets 150,000 mm^3, K 3.8 mEq/L, Na 140 mEq/L. An electrocardiogram (ECG, EKG) shows normal sinus rhythm. A kidneys, ureters, and bladder (KUB) abdominal X-ray is done, and she will have an esophagogastroduodenoscopy (EGD) at 7:00 A.M. the next day. She is admitted with the diagnosis of probable upper GI bleed. Ms. Winnie expresses concern to the nurse, "Do you think I'll be in the hospital long? I have been managing an important project for the past few months at the company I work for, and although my boss has been pretty understanding about me being out sick for the past few days, there is an important deadline coming up next week. Being in the hospital long may jeopardize my job." She is started on intravenous (IV) fluids of normal saline (NS) at 100 mL per hour. Pantoprazole continuous IV drip and prochlorperazine as needed for nausea and vomiting are prescribed. Ms. Winnie is to have strict monitoring of her intake and output and her vital signs assessed every two hours. She will be on bed rest. Her stools are to be tested for occult blood. She will have a complete blood count (CBC) assessed every six hours.

Results of the KUB are reported as a nonspecific gas pattern with moderate amount of stool throughout the colon with no acute abnormality noted. The EGD reveals a normal duodenum with no vascular anomalies, ulceration, or inflammation. There is a normal appearing gastric mucosa with no erosive changes, ulcer, or mass. A small Mallory-Weiss tear is noted.

Questions

1. The nurse asks Ms. Winnie if she takes any medications at home. Ms. Winnie states, "I take Ortho Tri-Cyclen once a day and I was taking Advil three to four times a day for the aches and pains of being sick." Should the nurse suggest to the health care provider that these two medications be included in Ms. Winnie's admission orders?

2. Identify four nursing diagnoses that are appropriate for Ms. Winnie upon admission.

3. Which lab results are abnormal and what is the significance of the abnormal results in Ms. Winnie's case?

4. Distinguish between the characteristics of upper and lower GI bleeding.

5. It is 1:00 A.M. and Ms. Winnie is settled into her room on the nursing unit. She asks the nurse, "Do you have some saltine crackers and ginger ale to try and help settle my stomach?" Should the nurse give Ms. Winnie something to eat?

6. The nurse recognizes the scenario in Question 5 as a teaching opportunity. How might the nurse explain why an EGD has been prescribed for Ms. Winnie and what she can expect during the procedure?

7. What are the nursing responsibilities after Ms. Winnie has the EGD and returns to her room?

8. Discuss the Mallory-Weiss tear found during Ms. Winnie's EGD. What is a Mallory-Weiss tear? What are the common symptoms of a Mallory-Weiss tear and what causes it?

9. Which factors determine if blood products will be administered to a client with GI tract bleeding secondary to a Mallory-Weiss tear?

Questions (continued)

10. If a transfusion is needed and Ms. Winnie's blood type is A positive, what are compatible blood types? Explain why a person can only receive compatible blood types.

11. Although unlikely with a Mallory-Weiss tear, the nurse realizes that if Ms. Winnie's bleeding does not resolve, she may need a blood transfusion. The nurse has not administered blood in a while and reviews the agency policy and procedure. Place the following ten steps of administering a blood transfusion in the proper order.

- Monitor vital signs per agency policy.
- Obtain blood products from the blood bank, keeping in mind that packed blood red cells (PRBC) transfusions should be completed within four hours of removal from refrigeration.
- Remain with the client during the first fifteen to thirty minutes of the transfusion (infusion of the first 50 ml of blood product) to assess for adverse reactions.
- Administer the blood product using appropriate filter tubing. Filters remove aggregates and possible contaminants. If blood is to be diluted, use only normal saline.
- Verify the medical prescription for type of blood product, dose, and transfusion time.
- Discontinue the transfusion when complete and dispose of the bag and tubing properly.

- Document type of blood product infused, time of infusion, and any adverse reactions.
- Obtain venous access with a larger-bore needle (19-gauge).
- Assess baseline vital signs, urine output, skin color, and history of transfusion reactions.
- With another registered nurse, verify the client by name and identification number, check blood product compatibility, and note expiration time. Do not use the client's room number as a form of client identification.

12. Later in the shift, the nurse is looking through Ms. Winnie's chart and comments to herself, "I think I may have reviewed the policy and procedure book for nothing." Why does the nurse believe she may not need to know how to administer blood to Ms. Winnie after all?

13. Which aspects of Ms. Winnie's plan of care could the registered nurse assign to assistive nursing personnel such as a certified nursing assistant (CNA)?

14. Should Ms. Winnie be concerned about her job? What do you anticipate will be her length of stay in the hospital?

15. If it is determined that Ms. Winnie has a bacterial infection and she is discharged with a prescription for an antibiotic, what teaching is appropriate regarding the use of an antibiotic with an oral contraceptive?

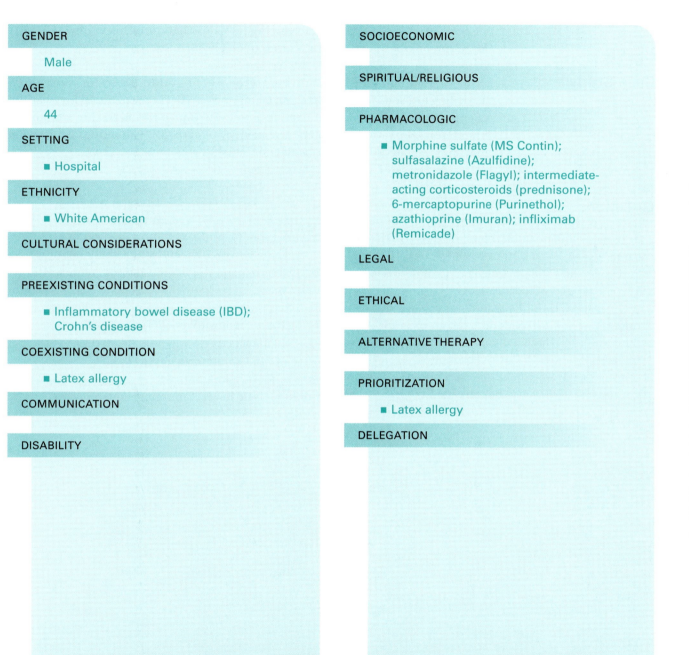

GENDER

Male

AGE

44

SETTING

- Hospital

ETHNICITY

- White American

CULTURAL CONSIDERATIONS

PREEXISTING CONDITIONS

- Inflammatory bowel disease (IBD); Crohn's disease

COEXISTING CONDITION

- Latex allergy

COMMUNICATION

DISABILITY

SOCIOECONOMIC

SPIRITUAL/RELIGIOUS

PHARMACOLOGIC

- Morphine sulfate (MS Contin); sulfasalazine (Azulfidine); metronidazole (Flagyl); intermediate-acting corticosteroids (prednisone); 6-mercaptopurine (Purinethol); azathioprine (Imuran); infliximab (Remicade)

LEGAL

ETHICAL

ALTERNATIVE THERAPY

PRIORITIZATION

- Latex allergy

DELEGATION

MODERATE

THE DIGESTIVE SYSTEM

Level of difficulty: Moderate

Overview: This case requires the nurse to differentiate between the characteristics of Crohn's disease and ulcerative colitis. Treatment options for Crohn's disease are reviewed. The nurse must provide safe care for a client with a latex allergy.

Client Profile

Mr. Cummings is a 44-year-old male admitted with lower right quadrant abdominal pain, nausea, and vomiting for four days. His past medical history is significant for inflammatory bowel disease (IBD) with Crohn's disease. The health care provider suspects Mr. Cummings is experiencing an exacerbation of his Crohn's disease. Mr. Cummings is scheduled for a series of diagnostic tests.

Case Study

Prior to Mr. Cummings's admission to the nursing unit, his room is prepared according to a latex-free protocol. Mr. Cummings is NPO in preparation for a barium enema, a colonoscopy, and to rest his bowel. The nurse caring for Mr. Cummings has identified pain management as a priority of care. Mr. Cummings is receiving morphine sulfate (MS Contin) with good effect.

Questions

1. What is inflammatory bowel disease (IBD)? Discuss the incidence and prevalence of IBD.

2. Discuss how the physiology of Crohn's disease differs from that of ulcerative colitis.

3. Briefly discuss the manifestations that are common to both Crohn's disease and ulcerative colitis and then discuss the manifestations that are characteristic of each disease.

4. Discuss the treatment options the health care provider will consider to help treat a Crohn's disease

exacerbation. Consider common medications prescribed, activity, diet, and surgical interventions.

5. Briefly explain the manifestations characteristic of the three types of latex reactions.

6. What precautions should the nurse take when caring for a client with an allergy to latex?

7. Explain why the hospital dietician should be aware of Mr. Cummings's allergy to latex.

8. List five potential nursing diagnoses the nurse should include in Mr. Cummings's plan of care.

Mrs. Bennett

GENDER

Female

AGE

63

SETTING

- Hospital

ETHNICITY

- White American

CULTURAL CONSIDERATIONS

PREEXISTING CONDITIONS

- Malabsorption syndrome (celiac disease); chronic wounds; pancreatitis with a pancreatic resection; depression

COEXISTING CONDITION

- Stage III coccyx pressure ulcer

COMMUNICATION

DISABILITY

- Has been on disability for the past five years

SOCIOECONOMIC

- Cared for in a nursing home for the past five years

SPIRITUAL/RELIGIOUS

PHARMACOLOGIC

- Allergy to erythromycin, tetracycline, tape, pneumococcal polysaccharide (pneumonia) vaccine

LEGAL

ETHICAL

ALTERNATIVE THERAPY

PRIORITIZATION

DELEGATION

- Collaboration with dietician and assistive nursing personnel

THE DIGESTIVE SYSTEM

Level of difficulty: Difficult

Overview: This case requires the nurse to consider the holistic effects of malabsorption syndrome on the client's health and quality of life. Symptoms of nutrient deficiencies are reviewed. The impact of poor nutrition on wound healing is discussed. The nurse must be attentive to the safety risks specific to this client. Priority nursing diagnoses are identified.

DIFFICULT

Client Profile

Mrs. Bennett is a 63-year-old woman with a history of malabsorption syndrome secondary to celiac disease. She is 5 foot 6 inches tall and weighs 100 pounds. She arrives in the emergency department from a nursing home with an elevated temperature and a decreased blood pressure and heart rate from her baseline. Her oxygen saturation is 89% on room air. She has a stage III pressure ulcer on her coccyx.

Case Study

Laboratory tests in the emergency department reveal Mrs. Bennett's white blood cell (WBC) count is 12,000 cells/mm^3, red blood cell (RBC) count is 3.16 million/mm^3, hemoglobin (Hgb) 8.9 g/dL, hematocrit (Hct) 25.7%, mean cell (or corpuscular) volume (MCV) 70.8 μm^3, mean cell (or corpuscular) hemoglobin (MCH) 20 pg, ferritin 7 mg/L, iron (Fe) 30 μg/L, total iron binding capacity (TIBC) 496 μg/dL, and transferrin 195 mg/dL. Her potassium (K$^+$) is 1.7 mEq/L, sodium (Na^{2+}) 128 mEq/L, chloride (Cl$^-$) 79 mmol/L, calcium (Ca^{2+}) 7.8 mg/dL, and protein 4.0 g/dL. Mrs. Bennett is admitted to the telemetry unit. She is placed on 4 liters of oxygen by nasal cannula. Her oxygen saturation improves to 96%. A regular diet is prescribed, with strict intake and output documentation and calorie counts. Because she will be primarily on bed rest, compression boots, graduated compression stockings (TEDs), and heel protectors are prescribed. Her dressing change documentation for the wound on her coccyx indicates that during each shift, the wound is to be gently irrigated with 250 mL of normal saline (NS), Mesalt rope moistened with NS is to be packed in the wound and in the areas of undermining, and then the entire wound is to be covered with Mesalt gauze dressings.

Questions

1. A colleague is not familiar with malabsorption syndrome. How would you explain what this condition is?

2. Intrigued, the colleague asks, "How would you know if you had malabsorption? What are the symptoms?" How would you answer?

3. If Mrs. Bennett were to have a deficiency of each of the following nutrients, what symptoms might she experience?

  1. calcium
  2. magnesium
  3. iron
  4. folic acid
  5. protein
  6. niacin (nicotinic acid)
  7. vitamin A (Retinol)
  8. vitamin B$_1$ (thiamine)
  9. vitamin B$_2$ (riboflavin)
  10. vitamin B$_{12}$
  11. vitamin C (ascorbic acid)
  12. vitamin D
  13. vitamin K

4. What would the nurse expect to find during assessment of Mrs. Bennett's HEENT (head, eyes, ears, nose, and throat), skin, abdomen, and extremities?

5. The nurse assesses Mrs. Bennett for Trousseau's and Chvostek's sign. What is the nurse looking for and if positive, what do these signs indicate?

6. The nurse is concerned that a regular diet is prescribed for Mrs. Bennett. The nurse calls Mrs. Bennett's health care provider to discuss the concern and suggest an alternate diet. What foods are allowed on a regular diet and what type of diet will the nurse suggest instead?

7. The nurse calls the dietician to discuss the scheduling of Mrs. Bennett's meals. What type of scheduling will the nurse suggest?

8. Why has Mrs. Bennett been admitted to a telemetry unit?

9. Intravenous (IV) potassium chloride is prescribed. Should the initial dose be administered as an IV push ("bolus dose") to help begin to correct

Questions (continued)

Mrs. Bennett's critically low potassium (K⁺) level of 1.7 mEq/L? Explain your answer.

10. Before hanging Mrs. Bennett's potassium, the nurse asks the assistive nursing personnel what Mrs. Bennett's urine output has been during the shift. Why is the nurse concerned about the client's urine output?

11. A type & cross match of two units of packed red blood cells (PRBC) has been added to Mrs. Bennett's medical treatment plan. Explain what it means to "type & cross match" and the rationale for including a PRBC transfusion in Mrs. Bennett's plan.

12. Mrs. Bennett says to the nurse "The other day I overheard my doctor tell someone I had nontropical sprue. As much as I wish that I was on a tropical vacation somewhere and not in the hospital, there is nothing warm and relaxing about what I have. What was he talking about?" Explain which disease the health care provider was discussing.

13. Briefly explain the significance of Mrs. Bennett's history of pancreatitis with a pancreatic resection to her present condition.

14. Which factors for proper wound healing are inadequate in Mrs. Bennett's case?

15. Mrs. Bennett has a prescription to obtain a wound culture during the next dressing change. Should the nurse obtain the wound sample before or after irrigating the wound with normal saline? Explain your answer.

16. Provide a rationale for including compression boots, graduated compression stockings (TEDs), and heel protectors in Mrs. Bennett's plan of care.

17. What must the nurse keep in mind when gathering supplies to do Mrs. Bennett's dressing change?

18. Identify five nursing diagnoses appropriate for Mrs. Bennett's plan of care. List the diagnoses in order of priority.

19. Which of Mrs. Bennett's allergies is of greatest concern and why?

20. Discuss the impact that a chronic illness has on a person's quality of life.

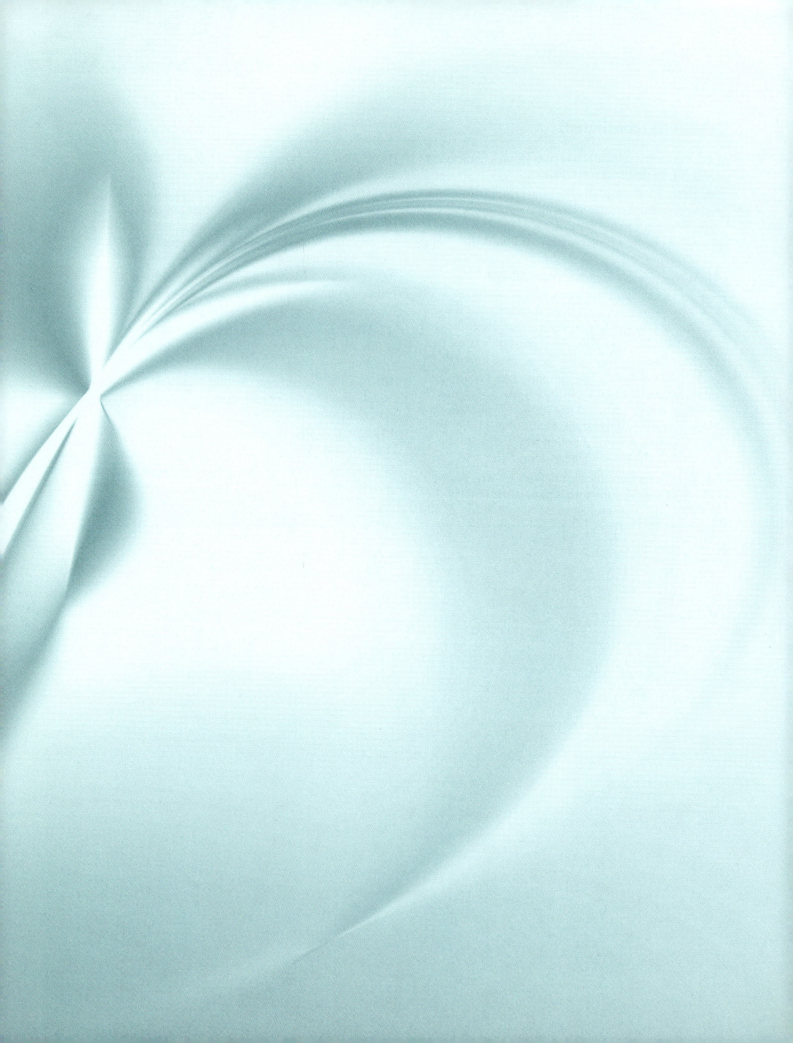

PART SEVEN

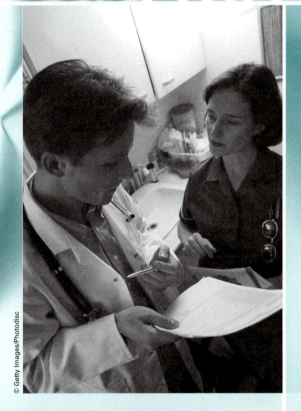

© Getty Images/Photodisc

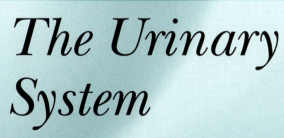

The Urinary System

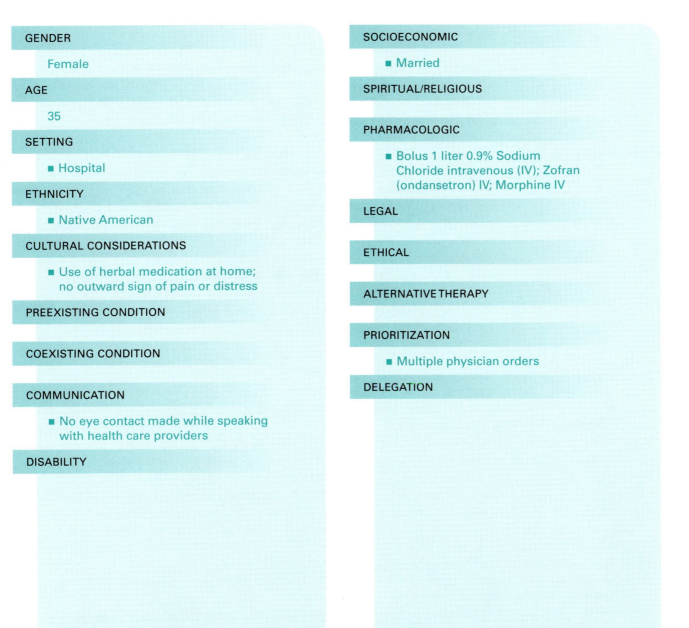

GENDER

Female

AGE

35

SETTING

- Hospital

ETHNICITY

- Native American

CULTURAL CONSIDERATIONS

- Use of herbal medication at home; no outward sign of pain or distress

PREEXISTING CONDITION

COEXISTING CONDITION

COMMUNICATION

- No eye contact made while speaking with health care providers

DISABILITY

SOCIOECONOMIC

- Married

SPIRITUAL/RELIGIOUS

PHARMACOLOGIC

- Bolus 1 liter 0.9% Sodium Chloride intravenous (IV); Zofran (ondansetron) IV; Morphine IV

LEGAL

ETHICAL

ALTERNATIVE THERAPY

PRIORITIZATION

- Multiple physician orders

DELEGATION

MODERATE

THE URINARY SYSTEM

Level of Difficulty: Moderate

Overview: The nurse must provide care for a 35-year-old female client with renal calculi. Coordination of care related to laboratory/diagnostic tests and IV medications will be discussed. Cultural considerations of caring for a Native American client are addressed. Priority nursing diagnoses are listed.

Client Profile

Mrs. Condiff is a 35-year-old female who presents to the emergency department with the chief complaint of severe right sided flank pain which began one day ago. She reports feeling nauseated and has vomited once today. Mrs. Condiff does not show any outward appearance of pain but is having some difficulty sitting still. She states, "I feel the need to constantly walk around." Upon further questioning, the client reveals a history of dysuria, urgency, and frequency of urination. As the nurse obtains a history, she notes that the client has no facial grimace and is not making eye contact. The client states, "I am sorry to come in with this pain, I have tried to treat it at home with Creeping Charlie but it just did not help."

Case Study

Nursing assessment findings include pale, moist skin, costovertebral tenderness, and restlessness. Her vital signs are blood pressure 142/90, pulse 110, respirations 22, and temperature of 99.8°F (37.7°C) Oxygen saturation is 98% on room air. The emergency physician evaluates Mrs. Condiff and orders the following: (a) urinalysis, strain all urine, (b) white blood count (WBC), (c) comprehensive metabolic panel (CMP), (d) intravenous pyelogram (IVP), (e) 1 liter 0.9% Sodium Chloride bolus, (f) Morphine 4mg IV, and (g) Zofran (ondansetron) 4mg IV. No physician orders have yet been implemented. The emergency physician informs the nurse that he suspects renal calculi to be the cause of this client's pain. Upon further assessment, the physician reports that the client has a family history of renal calculi. Mrs. Condiff rates the pain at a 9 on a 0-10 pain scale.

Questions

1. Mrs. Condiff asks the nurse, "What are renal calculi" Briefly explain what renal calculi are and how they are formed.

2. Identify at least 3 risk factors for renal calculi formation.

3. How should the nurse prioritize the physician orders above? Discuss which physician orders should be carried out first and the rationale for how you prioritized the orders.

4. Zofran and morphine have been ordered by the physician. Discuss the pharmacological classification of each of these medications, the rate at which they will be administered, and how the nurse will evaluate their effectiveness.

5. An IVP diagnostic test was ordered. What is the purpose of this test and what will the nurse do to prepare the client?

6. The physician has ordered that the urine needs to be strained. Discuss what straining the urine entails and why it is done.

7. Discuss the indication for the WBC, a CMP, and urinalysis ordered for this client.

8. In order to provide holistic client care, the nurse must be aware of cultural considerations. Using the information provided in regard to Mrs. Condiff, discuss how the nurse could incorporate culturally relevant care.

9. Discuss typical treatment options for renal calculi.

10. List five pertinent nursing diagnoses for Mrs. Condiff.

11. Discuss ways in which Mrs. Condiff can prevent further formation of renal calculi.

GENDER

Female

AGE

56

SETTING

- Hospital

ETHNICITY

- Hispanic

CULTURAL CONSIDERATIONS

PREEXISTING CONDITIONS

- Motor vehicle crash (MVC) eight weeks ago with no injury; depression

COEXISTING CONDITIONS

- Suicide attempt; metabolic acidosis

COMMUNICATION

DISABILITY

SOCIOECONOMIC

- Financial difficulties secondary to divorce five years ago; nonsmoker

SPIRITUAL/RELIGIOUS

PHARMACOLOGIC

- 4-methylpyrazole (Fomepizole; Antizol); pyridoxine hydrochloride (Vitamin B_6); thiamine (Vitamin B_1); succinylcholine chloride (Anectine); levalbuterol (Xopenex); lorazepam (Ativan); propofol (Diprivan, Disoprofol); etomidate

LEGAL

ETHICAL

ALTERNATIVE THERAPY

PRIORITIZATION

- Medical stabilization

DELEGATION

THE URINARY SYSTEM

Level of difficulty: Difficult

Overview: This case addresses the medical consequences of a failed suicide attempt. The nurse's understanding of the effects of ingesting ethylene glycol (antifreeze) is essential for prioritizing care, interpreting lab and arterial blood gas results, and identifying the purpose of prescribed medications.

Client Profile

Ms. Jimenez is a 56-year-old woman who has been having financial difficulties since her divorce five years ago. She was recently involved in a motor vehicle crash (MVC) in which she drove over a curb and hit a telephone pole. She did not sustain any significant injuries in the MVC. Today, Ms. Jimenez's daughter Maria returned home at 8:00 P.M. to find Ms. Jimenez sitting on the floor with a decreased level of consciousness. Maria was able to shake her mother awake. With slurred speech, Ms. Jimenez told her daughter that she drank three large glasses of antifreeze (ethylene glycol) at around 7:00 P.M. Maria called 911 and emergency medical services transported Ms. Jimenez to the local emergency department.

Case Study

Upon arrival to the emergency department, Ms. Jimenez is afebrile with a rectal temperature of 97°F (36.1°C). Her other vital signs are blood pressure 135/85, pulse 68, and respiratory rate 24. Her initial arterial blood gases (ABGs) on a 15 liters per minute non-rebreather revealed a pH of 7.19, partial pressure of carbon dioxide (PaCO$_2$) of 13 mmHg, partial pressure of oxygen (PaO$_2$) of 359 mmHg, bicarbonate (HCO$_3$$^-$) of 5 mEq/L, and oxygen (O$_2$) saturation of 100%. Ms. Jimenez is sedated in the emergency department using etomidate. She is intubated and put on a mechanical ventilator. A Foley catheter is inserted. She receives succinylcholine chloride, lorazepam, and propofol. Her oxygen saturation is 92% on an FIO$_2$ (fraction of inspired oxygen) of 70%. The health care provider's physical examination reveals no abnormal findings. The neurological exam is deferred because Ms. Jimenez is intubated and sedated. An electrocardiogram (ECG, EKG) shows that Ms. Jimenez is in a normal sinus rhythm. A chest X-ray (CXR) shows no infiltrate and proper endotracheal tube placement.

A urinalysis shows a specific gravity of 1.010, a small amount of occult blood, 3 to 5 white blood cells per high-power field (HPF), a few bacteria per HPF, and a moderate amount of uric acid crystals and urine calcium oxalate crystals. A urine culture & colony count was negative (no growth). Her blood alcohol level is less than 10 mg/dL. Her ethylene glycol level is 36 mg/dL. Her complete blood count (CBC) is within normal limits except for a mean cell volume (MCV) of 79.2 μm^3. Troponin level is 0 ng/mL, creatine kinase (CK) is 182 U/L, and creatine kinase cardiac isoenzyme (CK-MB) is within normal limits (WNL). Serum osmolality is 392 mOsm/Kg. Her electrolytes are WNL except for a serum bicarbonate of 7 mEq/L. She has an anion gap of 29 mEq/L, blood urea nitrogen (BUN) of 25 mg/dL, and creatinine of 1.4 mg/dL. Her liver function tests are WNL.

Ms. Jimenez is admitted to the intensive care unit (ICU) and prescribed intravenous (IV) fluids of normal saline with 2 ampules of bicarbonate at 125 mL per hour. The medications prescribed for her include 4-methylpyrazole IV every 12 hours, thiamine 100 mg IM, and levalbuterol treatments. Lab work prescribed includes CBC, electrolytes, ethylene glycol levels, basic metabolic panel (BMP), creatinine level, acetone level, and urinalysis.

In the ICU at the bedside, a Quinton dialysis catheter is surgically inserted in the right internal jugular vein for emergency dialysis and placement of the Quinton catheter is confirmed by CXR.

Questions

1. What is ethylene glycol? What products contain ethylene glycol?

2. Discuss the potential effects of ingesting ethylene glycol (antifreeze).

3. What is a "half-life"? Explain the half-life of ethylene glycol and how ethylene glycol is cleared from the body.

4. Ms. Jimenez's ethylene glycol level is 36 mg/dL. What is the lethal dose of ethylene glycol?

5. Discuss the rationale for why Ms. Jimenez is receiving 4-methylpyrazole. What is a drawback of this medication?

6. If 4-methylpyrazole is not available, what is the next most effective treatment for ethylene glycol poisoning? Discuss how this treatment is administered and what should be monitored during administration.

7. If Maria had come home earlier and Ms. Jimenez was found within half an hour of drinking the antifreeze, what three interventions could have been considered to decrease the progression of the toxic effects of the ethylene glycol?

8. Briefly describe the indication for each of the following medications Ms. Jimenez received during her initial medical treatment: thiamine, succinylcholine chloride, levalbuterol, lorazepam, propofol, and etomidate.

9. Why were intravenous (IV) fluids of normal saline with 2 ampules of bicarbonate at 125 mL per hour prescribed as part of the medical management of Ms. Jimenez?

10. Complete an analysis of Ms. Jimenez's initial arterial blood gas (ABG) results while on 15 liters of oxygen via non-rebreather. Are her ABG's consistent with those expected for a person with an ethylene glycol overdose?

11. Why was Ms. Jimenez intubated and placed on a mechanical ventilator?

12. Ms. Jimenez is on a mechanical ventilator set on assist-control of 14, respiratory rate of 28, volume 650, oxygen 40%, and a PEEP of 5. What does each ventilator setting indicate?

13. The respiratory rate on a mechanical ventilator is usually set between 10 and 14 breaths per minute. Why is the rate for Ms. Jimenez set at 28 breaths per minute?

14. Which of Ms. Jimenez's laboratory results below are most significant in the determination of a diagnosis of ethylene glycol poisoning?

- Urinalysis: specific gravity of 1.010, small amount of occult blood, 3 to 5 white blood cells per HPF, a few bacteria per HPF, and a moderate amount of uric acid crystals and urine calcium oxalate crystals.
- Urine culture & colony count was negative (no growth)
- Serum osmolality is 392 mOsm/Kg
- Bicarbonate of 7 mEq/L
- Anion gap of 29 mEq/L
- BUN of 25 mg/dL
- Creatinine of 1.4 mg/dL

15. Explain how a Wood lamp could be used to help confirm the ingestion of ethylene glycol.

16. Briefly explain what Ms. Jimenez's troponin, CPK, and CK-MB indicate.

17. Why did Ms. Jimenez's prescribed laboratory tests include an assessment of her liver function?

18. What is a Quinton catheter and why was one inserted?

19. Prioritize three nursing diagnoses that are appropriate to include in Ms. Jimenez's plan of care.

Ms. Jimenez (Part 2)

GENDER

Female

AGE

56

SETTING

- Hospital

ETHNICITY

- Hispanic

CULTURAL CONSIDERATIONS

PREEXISTING CONDITIONS

- Motor vehicle crash (MVC) eight weeks ago with no injury; depression

COEXISTING CONDITION

- Suicide attempt with ethylene glycol (antifreeze) poisoning

COMMUNICATION

DISABILITY

SOCIOECONOMIC

- Financial difficulties secondary to divorce five years ago; nonsmoker

SPIRITUAL/RELIGIOUS

PHARMACOLOGIC

LEGAL

- Safety sitter

ETHICAL

ALTERNATIVE THERAPY

PRIORITIZATION

- Client safety

DELEGATION

- Psychiatric consult; social services

MODERATE

THE URINARY SYSTEM

Level of difficulty: Moderate

Overview: The client ingested ethylene glycol two days ago and has been medically stabilized. The long-term effects of ethylene glycol poisoning are discussed. The nurse is asked to explain the stages of acute renal failure and the function of hemodialysis. Collaborative resources to assist the client following discharge are identified.

Client Profile

Ms. Jimenez is a 56-year-old woman who has been having financial difficulties since her divorce five years ago. She was recently involved in a motor vehicle crash (MVC) in which she drove over a curb and hit a telephone pole. She did not sustain any significant injuries in the MVC. Two days ago, Ms. Jimenez's daughter Maria returned home at 8:00 P.M. to find Ms. Jimenez sitting on the floor with a decreased level of consciousness. Maria was able to shake her mother awake. With slurred speech, Ms. Jimenez told her daughter that she drank three large glasses of antifreeze (ethylene glycol) at around 7:00 P.M. Maria called 911 and emergency medical services transported Ms. Jimenez to the local emergency department.

Case Study

It is forty-eight hours after her arrival in the emergency department. Ms. Jimenez has undergone twelve hours of emergency dialysis, has been extubated, and is medically stable for transfer to a medical-surgical nursing unit. A safety sitter remains in Ms. Jimenez's room at all times. Ms. Jimenez is alert and oriented but has a flat affect. She is not remorseful for her actions and states, "I had hoped I would be successful this time." A psychiatrist sees Ms. Jimenez for a consultation. The psychiatric assessment reveals that she has been planning the poisoning for a few weeks. She states, "I was hoping I would die quickly and it would look like an accident." Ms. Jimenez states that she has made attempts in the past to overdose on medications. She did not seek care at the hospital when these suicide attempts were not successful. She has been depressed since divorcing her husband five years ago. Since her divorce, she has not paid taxes and there have been mounting financial bills with the Internal Revenue Service. As a result, her wages are being garnished (money is withheld from her paycheck and sent to a creditor). She reports, "On the outside I appear bright and upbeat but on the inside I am so lonely and sad and just don't want to go on anymore." She wonders how she will pay for her medical care now. "I had not planned on the poison not working and needing dialysis. I bet dialysis is expensive."

Questions

1. Explain acute renal failure (ARF).

2. Considering the conditions that cause ARF, which type of ARF is Ms. Jimenez experiencing?

3. What characteristics and laboratory data define the four phases of acute renal failure, and what is the approximate duration of each phase?

4. It has been four days since admission. According to the definitions provided in the response to question number 3, which phase of acute renal failure is Ms. Jimenez experiencing?

5. While the nurse is assessing the Quinton catheter insertion site, Ms. Jimenez asks what dialysis is and how long she will need to do it. Her initial dialysis treatment was twelve hours long and she is wondering if she will always have to be "hooked up" to the machine that long each time. How should the nurse respond?

6. On admission, Ms. Jimenez's creatinine was 1.4 mg/dL and her BUN was 25 mg/dL. Ms. Jimenez has repeat creatinine and BUN labs drawn two days after admission. The results are a creatinine of 4.7 mg/dL and a BUN of 24 mg/dL. A day later her creatinine is 8.5 mg/dL with a BUN of 57 mg/dL. Are these results getting better or worse since admission? Discuss why.

7. The following potassium values are reported: on admission, 3.6 mEq/L; forty-eight hours after admission, 4.0 mEq/L; and seventy-two hours after admission, 4.2 mEq/L. What potential cardiovascular change is of greatest concern to the nurse?

8. Identify five priority nursing diagnoses that are appropriate to include in Ms. Jimenez's plan of care.

9. Why has a safety sitter been included as part of Ms. Jimenez's plan of care?

10. What are two collaborative services to consider when planning Ms. Jimenez's discharge?

11. Discuss how Ms. Jimenez's recent MVC may relate to her current admission.

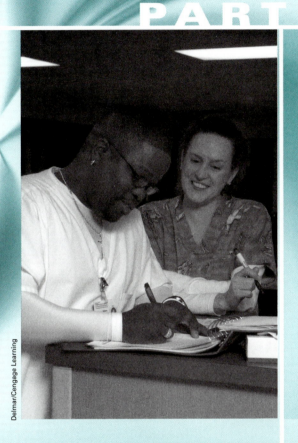

PART EIGHT

Delmar/Cengage Learning

The Endocrine/ Metabolic System

CASE STUDY 1

Mr. Rogers

GENDER

Male

AGE

91

SETTING

- Long-term care

ETHNICITY

- White American

CULTURAL CONSIDERATIONS

PREEXISTING CONDITIONS

- Benign prostatic hypertrophy (BPH); gout

COEXISTING CONDITION

COMMUNICATION

- Alert and oriented to person, place, and time

DISABILITY

SOCIOECONOMIC

- Long-term care resident for past nine years

SPIRITUAL/RELIGIOUS

PHARMACOLOGIC

- Colchicine; allopurinol (Alloprim); probenecid (*Benemid*); sulfinpyrazone (Anturane)

LEGAL

ETHICAL

ALTERNATIVE THERAPY

PRIORITIZATION

DELEGATION

- Nursing collaboration with the dietician

THE ENDOCRINE/METABOLIC SYSTEM

Level of difficulty: Easy

Overview: The client's symptoms are consistent with cellulitis. His history, however, necessitates consideration of the possibility of a recurrence of gout. The case requires the nurse to consider the defining characteristics of cellulitis and gout. Treatment options are discussed for the two possible diagnoses. Nursing priorities are considered following a definitive medical diagnosis.

Client Profile

Mr. Rogers is an 91-year-old resident of a long-term care facility who tells the nurse, "I have an ache in my right foot." He offers an explanation, suggesting, "I must have stepped on something or twisted my ankle. Maybe I got bit by a bug when I was outside yesterday." The nurse notes the medial aspect of Mr. Rogers's right ankle is reddened, slightly swollen, and warm. His temperature is within normal limits. He has a strong pedal pulse bilaterally.

Case Study

Mr. Rogers's ankle is X-rayed and there is no fracture noted. He has full range-of-motion of his right ankle and lower extremity, although the pain in his ankle increases with movement. A Doppler ultrasound rules out a deep vein thrombosis.

Questions

1. Prior to the Doppler ultrasound, how could the nurse explain this diagnostic procedure to prepare Mr. Rogers?

2. Define cellulitis and discuss its common manifestations.

3. Briefly explain what gout is and describe the causes of primary and secondary gout.

4. What are the common characteristics of each of the four stages of gout?

5. Explain what will facilitate a definitive diagnosis (cellulitis or gout) in Mr. Rogers's case.

6. If it is determined that Mr. Rogers has cellulitis, what treatments will the health care provider most likely prescribe?

7. If Mr. Rogers's symptoms are diagnosed as a recurrence of gout, what treatments will the health care provider most likely prescribe? Consider short- and long-term treatment.

8. The nurse collaborates with the dietician to adjust Mr. Rogers's diet to decrease his uric acid levels. Provide at least two examples of purine-containing foods and discuss appropriate fluid and alcohol intake to promote uric acid secretion.

9. Write a nursing diagnosis the nurse will consider adding to Mr. Rogers's plan of care upon learning the definitive diagnosis is gout.

CASE STUDY 2

Mr. Jenaro

GENDER

Male

AGE

61

SETTING

- Hospital

ETHNICITY

- Mexican American

CULTURAL CONSIDERATIONS

- Impact on diabetes education and disease management

PREEXISTING CONDITIONS

- Coronary artery disease (CAD); hypertension (HTN)

COEXISTING CONDITIONS

- Newly diagnosed diabetes; hyperglycemia

COMMUNICATION

- Spanish speaking; use of a medical interpreter

DISABILITY

SOCIOECONOMIC

- Smokes one pack of cigarettes per day; tobacco use for thirty-five years

SPIRITUAL/RELIGIOUS

PHARMACOLOGIC

- Regular insulin (Humulin R, Novolin R)

LEGAL

- Use of a medical interpreter

ETHICAL

- Use of a medical interpreter

ALTERNATIVE THERAPY

- Jerbero; curandera

PRIORITIZATION

DELEGATION

- Diabetes educator to assist with patient education

THE ENDOCRINE/METABOLIC SYSTEM

Level of difficulty: Moderate

Overview: This case requires the nurse to recognize the signs of hyperglycemia and convey an understanding of diabetes-related lab values. Type 1 and type 2 diabetes, complications of diabetes, and dietary guidelines are discussed. The nurse must consider the impact that culture may have on diabetes management. The nurse works with a diabetes educator to educate this newly diagnosed diabetic about blood glucose monitoring, medication administration, foot care, sick day management, and proper diet and exercise. The ethical and legal considerations of using an interpreter are addressed.

Client Profile

Mr. Jenaro is a 61-year-old Spanish-speaking man who presents to the emergency room with his wife Dolores. Mrs. Jenaro is also Spanish speaking, but understands some English. Mr. Jenaro complains of nausea and vomiting for two days and symptoms of confusion. His blood glucose is 796 mg/dL. Intravenous regular insulin (Novolin R) is prescribed and he is admitted for further evaluation. He will require teaching regarding his newly diagnosed diabetes.

Case Study

Mr. Jenaro is newly diagnosed with diabetes. His hemoglobin A1C is 10.3%. Mr. Jenaro is slightly overweight. He is 5 feet 10 inches tall and weighs 174 pounds (79 kg). He reports no form of regular exercise. He does not follow a special diet at home. He states, "I eat whatever Dolores puts in front of me. She is a good cook." For the past few months, Mrs. Jenaro has noticed that her husband "has been very thirsty and has been up and down to the bathroom a hundred times a day." Neither can recall how long it has been since these changes in Mr. Jenaro began. Dolores states, "It has been quite a while now. It just seems to be getting worse and worse."

Questions

1. The nurse does not speak Spanish. Discuss what the nurse should keep in mind to facilitate effective communication using an interpreter. What is the difference between the role of a medical "interpreter" and that of a medical "translator"?

2. Describe the following serum glucose tests used to help confirm the diagnosis of diabetes mellitus: casual, fasting, postprandial, and oral glucose tolerance test.

3. When evaluating Mr. Jenaro's postprandial result, what is important to consider regarding his age and tobacco use?

4. Explain what a hemoglobin A1C (HbA$_{1C}$) lab test tells the health care provider.

5. How might the nurse briefly explain what diabetes is in lay terms to Mr. and Mrs. Jenaro?

6. Explain the difference between type 1 diabetes and type 2 diabetes and who is at increased risk for developing each type. Based on this understanding, which type of diabetes does Mr. Jenaro have?

7. Discuss the prevalence of diabetes and the potential long-term complications of diabetes.

8. List five nursing diagnoses appropriate to consider for Mr. Jenaro.

9. Discuss Mr. and Mrs. Jenaro's learning needs. Consider the communication preferences of Mexican Americans.

10. Discuss the dietary recommendations for a diabetic based on the Diabetes Food Pyramid.

11. Discuss how culture may influence Mr. Jenaro's diabetes management in terms of food choices, diet and exercise, and use of an alternative health care provider.

12. Discuss the information the nurse and/or diabetes educator should include when teaching Mr. Jenaro about proper foot care.

13. Discuss the lifestyle considerations the nurse and/or diabetes educator should discuss with Mr. Jenaro and his wife.

14. Discuss what Mr. Jenaro should be taught about how to manage his diabetes on days that he is ill (e.g., if he were to have a stomach virus).

15. Mr. Jenaro meets his friends at a local bar once a week for a beer or two. What impact does alcohol have on a diabetic? Should he discontinue this social activity?

CASE STUDY 3

Mrs. Miller

GENDER

> Female

AGE

> 88

SETTING

- Hospital

ETHNICITY

- White American

CULTURAL CONSIDERATIONS

PREEXISTING CONDITIONS

- Heart failure (HF); hypothyroidism; gastroesophageal reflux disease (GERD); allergy to penicillin (PCN)

COEXISTING CONDITION

COMMUNICATION

DISABILITY

SOCIOECONOMIC

SPIRITUAL/RELIGIOUS

PHARMACOLOGIC

- Potassium chloride (KCl); pantoprazole sodium (Protonix); levothyroxine sodium (Synthroid); spironolactone (Aldactone); metoclopramide (Reglan); morphine sulfate (MS Contin)

LEGAL

ETHICAL

ALTERNATIVE THERAPY

PRIORITIZATION

DELEGATION

THE ENDOCRINE/METABOLIC SYSTEM

Level of difficulty: Difficult

Overview: This case discusses the diagnostic characteristics and treatment of acute pancreatitis. Use of the Ranson and Glasgow criteria assessment tools to determine disease severity is explained. Potential complications of acute pancreatitis are considered. The nurse educates the client about a scheduled diagnostic procedure to help reduce the client's anxiety. Safe administration of a medication via a nasogastric tube is ensured.

Client Profile

Mrs. Miller is an 88-year-old woman who presented with complaints of nausea, vomiting, and abdominal pain. Her vital signs on admission are temperature 99.6°F (37.6°C), blood pressure 113/82, pulse 84, and respiratory rate 20. Her laboratory tests reveal white blood cell count (WBC) 13,000/mm^3, potassium (K$^+$) 3.2 mEq/L, lipase 449 units/L, amylase 306 units/L, total bilirubin 3.4 mg/dL, direct bilirubin 2.2 mg/dL, aspartate aminotransferase (AST) 142 U/L, and alanine aminotransferase (ALT) 390 U/L. Physical examination reveals a distended abdomen that is very tender on palpation. Bowel sounds are present in all four quadrants, but hypoactive. Mrs. Miller is admitted with a diagnosis of acute pancreatitis. She will be kept nothing by mouth (NPO). Intravenous (IV) fluid of D51/2 NS with 40 mEq of potassium chloride (KCl) per liter at 100 mL per hour is prescribed. The health care provider prescribes continued administration of her preadmission medications, that is, pantoprazole sodium and levothyroxine sodium (in IV form because the client is NPO) and spironolactone (available in oral form), and adds the prescription of IV metoclopramide and morphine sulfate. A nasogastric (NG) tube is inserted and attached to low wall suction.

Case Study

Mrs. Miller's NG tube is draining yellow-brown drainage. Her pain is being managed effectively with IV morphine 4 mg every four hours. Mrs. Miller is anxious and has many questions for the nurse: "What is the test I am having done today? What is pancreatitis? Will I need to have surgery? Why did they put this tube in my nose? When will I be able to eat real food?"

Questions

1. Briefly explain acute pancreatitis and discuss its incidence.

2. Mrs. Miller's admitting diagnosis is acute pancreatitis. Can a person have chronic pancreatitis? If so, what is the incidence, and how would you define chronic pancreatitis?

3. Discuss the common clinical manifestations of acute pancreatitis.

4. Briefly discuss the diagnostic tests that help confirm the diagnosis of pancreatitis.

5. Identify the assessment findings in Mrs. Miller's case that are consistent with acute pancreatitis.

6. Identify the possible causes of acute pancreatitis. Discuss the physiology of the two major causes of acute pancreatitis in the United States, and note which individuals are at greatest risk.

7. The severity of an acute pancreatitis episode can be assessed using two tools: (1) Ranson/Imrie criteria and (2) modified Glasgow criteria. Describe each of these tools.

8. Briefly discuss the treatment options for pancreatitis, and explain why Mrs. Miller has an NG tube to low wall suction.

9. Discuss the complications that can arise if pancreatitis is not treated.

10. Evaluate Mrs. Miller's potassium level. Should the nurse question the health care provider's prescription for the diuretic spironolactone? Why or why not?

11. Because Mrs. Miller is NPO, the nurse must administer the oral spironolactone via the NG tube. Is it appropriate to crush this medication? Why or why not? What intervention should the nurse take following administration of the medication to facilitate absorption?

12. Which type of diet will Mrs. Miller advance to when her NPO status is discontinued? What types of liquids are allowed on this diet?

13. Identify the priority nursing diagnosis for Mrs. Miller's plan of care and two additional nursing diagnoses that the nurse should consider.

PART NINE

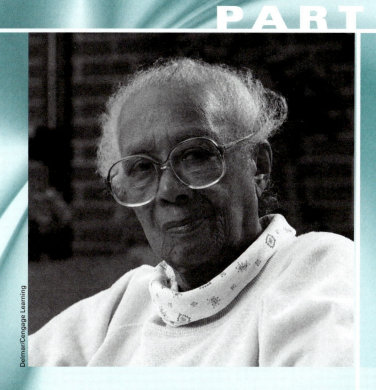

The Skeletal System

Mr. Mendes

GENDER

Male

AGE

81

SETTING

- Hospital

ETHNICITY

- Portuguese

CULTURAL CONSIDERATIONS

- Language barrier

PREEXISTING CONDITIONS

- Peripheral vascular disease (PVD); type 1 diabetes; below the knee amputation (BKA, B-K amputation) of left leg two weeks ago

COEXISTING CONDITION

- Left lower lobe pneumonia

COMMUNICATION

- Non-English speaking

DISABILITY

- Uses a wheelchair; needs assistance with activities of daily living (ADLs)

SOCIOECONOMIC

- Admitted from a rehabilitation health care center

SPIRITUAL/RELIGIOUS

PHARMACOLOGIC

LEGAL

- Use of a medical interpreter

ETHICAL

- Use of a medical interpreter

ALTERNATIVE THERAPY

PRIORITIZATION

DELEGATION

EASY

THE SKELETAL SYSTEM

Level of difficulty: Easy

Overview: This case challenges the nurse to identify strategies to help overcome a language barrier and form a therapeutic nurse–client relationship. Legal and ethical concerns regarding the use of an interpreter are considered. Stump care for the client with a recent amputation is discussed.

Client Profile

Mr. Mendes is an 81-year-old man who speaks only Portuguese. He is quite frail, weighing only 110 pounds. He had a below-the-knee amputation of his left leg two weeks ago. Mr. Mendes has been admitted to the hospital from a rehabilitation center with an acute change in mental status and diminished lung sounds in the left base. Mr. Mendes is diagnosed with left lower lobe pneumonia and antibiotic therapy is prescribed. The nurse assigned to care for Mr. Mendes does not speak Portuguese.

Case Study

Mr. Mendes requires complete assistance with activities of daily living (ADLs). A medical interpreter is not assigned to the nursing unit; but, if needed, the nurse can ask a Portuguese-speaking nursing staff member to help interpret what Mr. Mendes is trying to express. However, the nurse still must develop a way of communicating with Mr. Mendes so the nurse can assess Mr. Mendes's level of comfort, provide care, and identify any needs.

Questions

1. Briefly discuss the challenges of developing a nurse–client relationship when a language barrier exists between the client and nurse.

2. Explain the difference between a medical "interpreter" and a medical "translator."

3. Family members are often willing to interpret for the client and are more readily available. Discuss the use of medical interpreters and why, legally and ethically, family members (or friends of the client) are not the preferred interpreter(s).

4. Describe a therapeutic nurse–client relationship.

5. The nurse does not speak Portuguese. Discuss nonverbal strategies the nurse can implement to help develop a therapeutic relationship with Mr. Mendes.

6. Provide the most likely explanation for why Mr. Mendes presented with an acute change in mental status.

7. Briefly discuss how Mr. Mendes's past medical history relates to his below-the-knee leg amputation. What is the benefit of having a below-the-knee (B-K) amputation versus an above-the-knee (A-K) amputation?

8. The interpreter tells the nurse that Mr. Mendes would like the nurse to remove the bed linens from his left foot and raise his leg on pillows. He states, "My foot aches and maybe if you put it up it on some pillows will feel better." Provide a rationale for Mr. Mendes's request. Should the nurse elevate his stump on pillows as requested? Why or why not?

9. Mr. Mendes has not yet been fit for a prosthesis. The nurse provides care of his stump. Briefly discuss the nursing interventions involved in stump care. What outcome goals does the nurse hope to achieve through proper stump care?

10. List five nursing diagnoses appropriate to consider for Mr. Mendes's plan of care.

GENDER

Female

AGE

77

SETTING

- Hospital

ETHNICITY

- Black American

CULTURAL CONSIDERATIONS

- Age-related complications

PREEXISTING CONDITION

- Osteoporosis

COEXISTING CONDITION

- Recent fall

COMMUNICATION

DISABILITY

- Potential impact of a hip fracture on quality of life

SOCIOECONOMIC

- Lives at home

SPIRITUAL/RELIGIOUS

PHARMACOLOGIC

- Alendronate sodium (Fosamax)

LEGAL

ETHICAL

ALTERNATIVE THERAPY

PRIORITIZATION

DELEGATION

- Home safety assessment by the visiting nurse

THE SKELETAL SYSTEM

Level of difficulty: Easy

Overview: This case requires that the nurse consider appropriate pre- and postoperative nursing interventions for a client with a hip fracture. A new medication is prescribed and teaching is needed. Considerations for recovery related to the client's age as well as the safety of her home environment are discussed. The nurse is asked to prioritize appropriate nursing diagnoses for the client's postoperative plan of care.

Client Profile

Mrs. Damerae is a 77-year-old woman who was transported to the emergency department following a fall onto her right hip on a snowy morning. "I just wanted to check the mail. I was making my way down my front walk slowly. I had my good boots on. But there must have been ice under the snow and I slipped. It all happened so fast. I was up. I was down. And here I am."

Case Study

Physical exam reveals that Mrs. Damerae's right leg is shorter than her left leg and her right leg is externally rotated. There is bruising of her right hip. An X-ray confirms that Mrs. Damerae has an extracapsular fracture of the trochanter region of her right hip. Mrs. Damerae will have an open reduction of the fracture and internal fixation (ORIF) surgery the next morning.

Questions

1. Prior to surgery, the health care provider chooses to place Mrs. Damerae's right leg in Buck's extension (traction). Why is this intervention prescribed prior to surgery?

2. A trochanter roll is another option for Mrs. Damerae. What is a trochanter roll and how would it be useful?

3. How might Mrs. Damerae's age affect her hospitalization and recovery?

4. Briefly discuss how Mrs. Damerae's past medical history played a role in her injury.

5. Mrs. Damerae's surgeon informs her of the potential complications of hip surgery. Identify at least three complications the surgeon will address.

6. Prioritize five nursing diagnoses appropriate for Mrs. Damerae following surgery.

7. Explain how the nurse should move Mrs. Damerae in order to position her safely on her side to wash her back.

8. The nurse applies graduated compression stockings (TEDs) and sequential compression devices (SCDs) as prescribed. What is the rationale for these interventions?

9. Mrs. Damerae asks for assistance to the bathroom. The nurse checks to see that the appropriate equipment is available in the bathroom before assisting the client to ambulate. What is the nurse looking for in the bathroom?

10. Mrs. Damerae is assisted back to bed. She asks that the head of her bed be raised so she can read. How high should the head of the bed be raised and why?

11. Mrs. Damerae is seated in a reclining chair. What reminders will the nurse give Mrs. Damerae regarding positioning while sitting and why is positioning so important?

12. Identify the indications of a possible hip dislocation that the nurse should watch for.

13. If the nurse notices any of the above signs, discuss the appropriate action for the nurse to take.

14. Alendronate sodium is prescribed for Mrs. Damerae. What is the rationale for the use of alendronate sodium? Discuss the client education regarding proper administration to maximize the benefits of alendronate sodium and adverse effects.

15. Following discharge from a rehabilitation unit, a visiting nurse will provide follow-up care for Mrs. Damerae. On the first home visit, the nurse conducts a home safety assessment. Identify at least five components of a safe home environment.

Mr. Lourde

GENDER

Male

AGE

73

SETTING

- Hospital

ETHNICITY

- White American

CULTURAL CONSIDERATIONS

PREEXISTING CONDITIONS

- Left hip replacement two years ago; septic shock with left hip osteomyelitis last year with subsequent removal of the hip replacement prosthesis; allergies to meperidine hydrochloride (Demerol), morphine sulfate (MS Contin), and vancomycin hydrochloride (Vancocin)

COEXISTING CONDITION

COMMUNICATION

DISABILITY

SOCIOECONOMIC

SPIRITUAL/RELIGIOUS

PHARMACOLOGIC

- Linezolid (Zyvox); fondaparinux (Arixtra); hydrocodone bitartrate/acetaminophen (Vicodin); acetaminophen (Tylenol); docusate sodium (Colace)

LEGAL

ETHICAL

ALTERNATIVE THERAPY

PRIORITIZATION

DELEGATION

MODERATE

THE SKELETAL SYSTEM

Level of difficulty: Moderate

Overview: This case requires that the nurse understand the risk associated with postoperative wound infection following a hip replacement. The manifestations characteristic of osteomyelitis are discussed. The nurse must care for the surgical incision site with a daily dressing change and maintenance of a HemoVac drainage system. The client's prescribed medications are reviewed for purpose and potential adverse effects. The purpose and potential complications of a peripherally inserted central catheter (PICC) are explained.

Client Profile

Mr. Lourde is a 73-year-old man whose wife noticed a lump on his left hip that has increased in size over the past two weeks. The skin around the lump is red and swollen. Mr. Lourde complains of increasing discomfort in his left hip. His wife became concerned when he felt warm and his temperature was 101°F (38.3°C) so she brought him to the hospital. Mr. Lourde is diagnosed with an abscess of his left hip. A needle aspiration of the abscess reveals 30 mL of purulent exudate. Mr. Lourde is admitted for surgical incision and drainage of a suspected recurrence of osteomyelitis and for intravenous antibiotic therapy.

Case Study

A surgical incision and drainage is performed to remove necrotic tissue, sequestrum, and surrounding granulation tissue. A bacterial infection is identified as *Enterococcus faecalis*. The nurse reviews the client's kardex and notes the dressing change prescribed is a dry sterile dressing to the left hip daily with reinforcement as needed.

The nurse medicates Mr. Lourde with hydrocodone/acetaminophen (Vicodin) thirty minutes prior to the dressing change. While changing the hip dressing, the nurse notes there are seven intact sutures along the incision line, and a HemoVac drain is in place. Minimal drainage is noted at the incision site. The site is slightly swollen, but there are no signs of infection. The HemoVac has drained 30 mL of dark red blood. Mr. Lourde tolerates the dressing change with minimal discomfort. He is afebrile at 98°F (36.7°C).

Questions

1. Discuss the time frame within which signs of an infection at the site of a hip replacement usually occur. What possible complications are of concern when a client develops an infection at the site of a hip replacement?

2. Discuss the pathophysiology of osteomyelitis. Include an explanation of a sequestrum, involucrum, and Brodie's abscess.

3. Discuss the clinical manifestations of osteomyelitis.

4. The health care provider suspects a recurrence of Mr. Lourde's osteomyelitis. How will the health care provider confirm this diagnosis?

5. Discuss the treatment options if Mr. Lourde has osteomyelitis of his left hip.

6. Mr. Lourde will require at least three to eight weeks of high-dose intravenous antibiotic therapy. The health care provider has requested that a PICC be inserted. Explain what a PICC is and the potential complications associated with this device.

7. What information should be included in the nurse's documentation of the dressing change?

8. Explain why the nurse does not document the stage of the left hip wound.

9. Write two expected outcomes for the duration of time that a HemoVac drainage reservoir system is in place. How often should the nurse empty the drain and how will the nurse ensure that the system is working correctly to drain the incision site?

10. Each of the medications below is prescribed for Mr. Lourde. For each, provide the therapeutic drug classification and discuss the purpose of the medication for Mr. Lourde and potential adverse effect(s) that the nurse should monitor.

    1. Linezolid
    2. Fondaparinux
    3. Hydrocodone bitartrate/acetaminophen
    4. Acetaminophen
    5. Docusate sodium

11. Help the nurse generate three appropriate nursing diagnoses for Mr. Lourde.

PART TEN

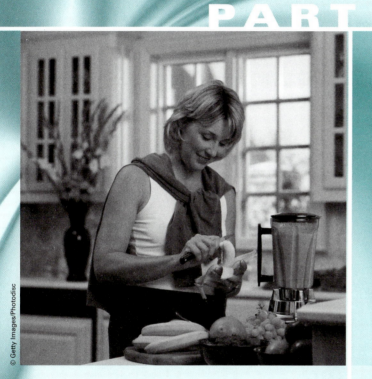

The Muscular System

CASE STUDY 1

Mr. O'Brien

GENDER

Male

AGE

81

SETTING

- Hospital

ETHNICITY

- White American

CULTURAL CONSIDERATIONS

PREEXISTING CONDITIONS

- Atrial fibrillation (AFib); syncope; peripheral vascular disease (PVD)

COEXISTING CONDITION

- Hypotension

COMMUNICATION

DISABILITY

- Ambulates with a walker and one assist

SOCIOECONOMIC

- Resides in a long-term nursing care facility; financial and social implications of fall-related injuries

SPIRITUAL/RELIGIOUS

PHARMACOLOGIC

- Oxycodone/acetaminophen 5/325 (Percocet)

LEGAL

- Fall precautions; incident report (occurrence or variance report); restraints

ETHICAL

ALTERNATIVE THERAPY

PRIORITIZATION

DELEGATION

- Nursing assistant's role

THE MUSCULAR SYSTEM

Level of difficulty: Easy

Overview: This case requires the nurse to identify appropriate interventions upon learning that a client has fallen. The nurse is asked to discuss fall precautions and proper documentation of a client safety incident. The use of a restraint is considered. The nurse must also assess the client for orthostatic (postural) hypotension. The incidence of falls, injuries resulting, fall-related deaths, financial and social implications, and need for long-term care following a fall are reviewed.

Client Profile

Mr. O'Brien is an alert and oriented 81-year-old man admitted to the hospital with complaints of dizziness and syncope. His blood pressure (BP) on admission is 80/43. At the long-term nursing care facility where he lives, he ambulated with a walker independently but, since his episode of syncope, he has complained of weakness and needs another person to assist while walking as a fall precaution.

Case Study

Mr. O'Brien is admitted with prescriptions that include assessment of orthostatic vital signs every shift and fall precautions. The nurse explains to Mr. O'Brien how to use the call light and instructs him to call before getting out of bed so that someone can assist him with ambulation. The nurse completes a set of orthostatic vital signs. His orthostatic vital signs are lying: BP = 120/84, heart rate (HR) = 73; sitting: BP = 114/73, HR = 83; standing: BP = 96/61, HR = 92. When the assessment of orthostatics is complete, Mr. O'Brien is settled in bed. The nurse raises two side rails at the head of the bed, and the bed alarm is turned on so that if Mr. O'Brien tries to get out of bed without assistance, an alarm will notify staff.

Later in the shift, Mr. O'Brien's bed alarm sounds. The nurse quickly goes to his room to find Mr. O'Brien lying on the floor on his right hip. He is alert and oriented and states, "I had to go to the bathroom. I know I should have called for help but the nurses are busy. I figured I could go myself. Only two more steps and I could have reached my walker. I just slipped is all." Immediately following his fall, Mr. O'Brien complains of pain in his right hip that is a "7" on a 0–10 pain scale. He describes the pain as a "dull ache" that is worse with movement of his right leg. His BP is 110/62, HR is 88, and respiratory rate (RR) is 16.

Questions

1. Which clients are at greatest risk for falls in the acute care setting? Consider physiological and environmental risk factors for falls.

2. Identify seven areas of a fall risk assessment.

3. Discuss the initial nursing interventions when the nurse enters Mr. O'Brien's room and finds him lying on the floor.

4. Discuss who should be notified about Mr. O'Brien's fall and what type of documentation is needed regarding the incident.

5. What test(s) will the health care provider most likely prescribe because Mr. O'Brien is complaining of pain in his right hip?

6. The nurse double checks to see that appropriate fall precautions are in place. Identify ten measures to help prevent falls in older adults.

7. What can the nursing assistant do to help in maintaining Mr. O'Brien's safety?

8. The nurse must complete an incident report. Discuss the purpose of an incident report and list the elements/type of data to address when completing this report.

9. Mr. O'Brien was assisted back to bed with a Hoyer lift and two assists. His vital signs remained within his baseline throughout the remainder of the shift and he is afebrile. An X-ray of his right hip was negative for a fracture. There is no physical deformity of the right hip or other injuries apparent, but a moderate amount of ecchymosis of his right hip that extends around to his lower back and right upper buttock is noted. His health care provider, Dr. Sutton, prescribed one tablet of oxycodone/acetaminophen 5/325 by mouth (PO) that decreased Mr. O'Brien's pain to a "2/10" within forty minutes of administration. He remains alert and oriented, continues on bed rest, and used the urinal once for 200 mL of clear yellow urine. The bed alarm is on, the call bell is in reach, and there are two side rails up. Mr. O'Brien has verbalized an understanding of how and when to use the call bell. Write a nursing progress note regarding the fall to enter into Mr. O'Brien's chart. Use the S.O.A.P.I.E. or Focus/D.A.R. method for writing a nursing note.

10. Provide a brief explanation of what orthostatic (postural) hypotension is and identify the blood pressure and heart rate values that define orthostatic (postural) hypotension.

Questions (continued)

11. Explain the steps of assessing orthostatic vital signs. From a lying to standing position, is Mr. O'Brien exhibiting signs of orthostatic hypotension based on the vital signs the nurse collected?

12. Identify Mr. O'Brien's predisposing risk factors for a fall.

13. The use of a vest restraint could be considered for Mr. O'Brien to prevent another fall. Define a *restraint* and provide examples of physical restraints and chemical restraints.

14. Discuss the risk of client injury associated with the use of restraints and the prescription requirements to implement restraints.

15. Identify five alternatives to using restraints.

16. Briefly address the following: (a) What is the incidence of falls and fall-related deaths in the older adult population? (b) Is there a difference in the incidence and mortality between men and women? If so, explain. (c) What are the common injuries that result from a fall? (d) What are the potential social implications for the older adult who has suffered a fall? (e) Describe the need for long-term care following a fall.

17. The most common fracture resulting from a fall is a hip fracture. Discuss the incidence of and mortality associated with a hip fracture, as well as the difference in the incidence of hip fractures between men and women.

18. What is a "HipSaver"?

19. Write an appropriate three-part nursing diagnosis to include in Mr. O'Brien's plan of care regarding his fall.

Mrs. Roberts

GENDER

Female

AGE

48

SETTING

- Primary care

ETHNICITY

- White American

CULTURAL CONSIDERATIONS

PREEXISTING CONDITIONS

- Gastroesophageal reflux disease (GERD); irritable bowel syndrome (IBS)

COEXISTING CONDITION

COMMUNICATION

DISABILITY

- Potential disability resulting from chronic illness

SOCIOECONOMIC

- Wife; mother of three children (ages 21, 19, and 16 years); employed as an elementary school teacher

SPIRITUAL/RELIGIOUS

PHARMACOLOGIC

- Pantoprazole sodium (Protonix); acetaminophen (Tylenol); lidocaine hydrochloride

LEGAL

ETHICAL

ALTERNATIVE THERAPY

- Complementary therapies for managing symptoms of fibromyalgia

PRIORITIZATION

DELEGATION

MODERATE

THE MUSCULAR SYSTEM

Level of difficulty: Moderate

Overview: The client has been recently diagnosed with fibromyalgia. This case requires the nurse to provide the client with information about her diagnosis. The impact of a chronic illness on the client's quality of life is considered.

Client Profile

Mrs. Roberts is a 48-year-old elementary school teacher and mother of three children. Her past medical history includes GERD, which is well controlled with daily pantoprazole (Protonix). She also has a history of irritable bowel syndrome. For the past three and a half years, she has experienced "incredible" exhaustion and arthritis-like symptoms that make her "hurt all over."

Case Study

Years of assessment and testing to rule out several diagnostic possibilities have finally resulted in the diagnosis of fibromyalgia. A follow-up appointment is scheduled at the primary care provider's office to discuss the diagnosis with Mrs. Roberts. Her husband accompanies her to the appointment.

Questions

1. How might the nurse explain what fibromyalgia is to Mr. and Mrs. Roberts? Include the prevalence of fibromyalgia in the United States and the diagnostic criteria.

2. What are the common manifestations of fibromyalgia?

3. Mrs. Roberts asks, "I live a healthy lifestyle. What caused me to get this?" How will the nurse respond?

4. Discuss the focus of care for the client with fibromyalgia.

5. Discuss interventions that may be suggested to help Mrs. Roberts manage her fibromyalgia.

Consider medications, exercise, rest, and alternative therapies.

6. Mr. Roberts asks, "How will fibromyalgia affect my wife's everyday life?" What are the potential quality-of-life changes that Mrs. Roberts may experience because of this chronic condition?

7. How can the nurse support Mrs. Roberts as she begins to cope with the news of this new diagnosis?

8. Generate at least three possible nursing diagnoses appropriate for Mrs. Roberts.

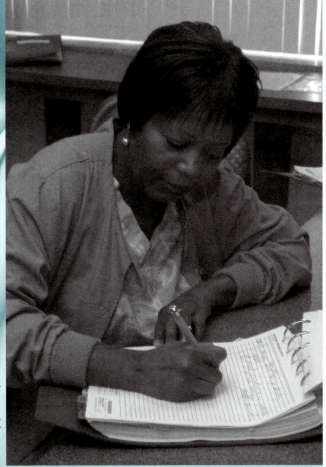

PART ELEVEN

Delmar/Cengage Learning

The Reproductive System

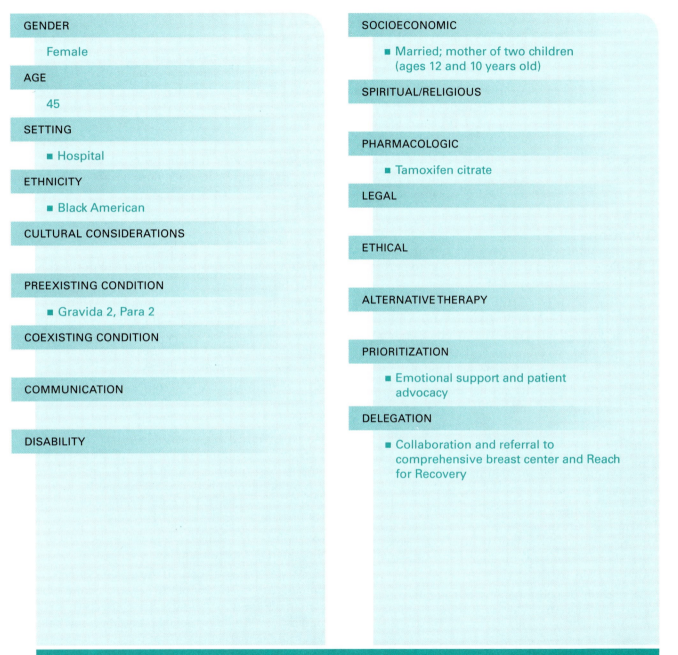

GENDER

Female

AGE

45

SETTING

- Hospital

ETHNICITY

- Black American

CULTURAL CONSIDERATIONS

PREEXISTING CONDITION

- Gravida 2, Para 2

COEXISTING CONDITION

COMMUNICATION

DISABILITY

SOCIOECONOMIC

- Married; mother of two children (ages 12 and 10 years old)

SPIRITUAL/RELIGIOUS

PHARMACOLOGIC

- Tamoxifen citrate

LEGAL

ETHICAL

ALTERNATIVE THERAPY

PRIORITIZATION

- Emotional support and patient advocacy

DELEGATION

- Collaboration and referral to comprehensive breast center and Reach for Recovery

EASY

THE REPRODUCTIVE SYSTEM

Level of difficulty: Easy

Overview: The client in this case requires nursing support during the diagnostic phase of breast cancer. Nursing care for the pre- and postoperative client is discussed. Priority nursing diagnoses in the postoperative period are identified. The use of tamoxifen after surgery is explained and the purpose of a port-a-cath device is reviewed. The nurse must provide discharge instructions and referral for ongoing rehabilitation and support.

Client Profile

Mrs. Whitney is a 45-year-old woman who noticed a lump in her left breast during her monthly breast self-exam two weeks ago. She made an appointment with her gynecologist who documents "a fixed round lump with irregular borders palpated in the upper outer quadrant of left breast at 2:00. Left axillary edema noted. There is symmetry of the breasts with no puckering or nipple discharge. The client denies pain." Mrs. Whitney began having her menstrual period at 10 years of age. She has two children, both of whom she breastfed for approximately twelve months. Mrs. Whitney's oldest sister died of breast cancer. Mrs. Whitney has a diagnostic mammogram and a fine-needle aspiration biopsy. It is determined that she has stage II breast cancer.

Case Study

Mrs. Whitney will have a lumpectomy with lymph node dissection (partial mastectomy). A Jackson-Pratt (JP) drain will be in place postoperatively. Following surgery, tamoxifen is prescribed.

Questions

1. Discuss the best time of the month to perform breast self-examination (BSE).

2. What factors placed Mrs. Whitney at greater risk for the development of breast cancer? Discuss the risk factors associated with Mrs. Whitney's ethnicity.

3. Mrs. Whitney's past medical history is "gravida 2, para 2." Explain what these terms indicate.

4. Discuss the priority nursing intervention prior to Mrs. Whitney's biopsy and immediately following diagnosis.

5. The nurse is teaching Mrs. Whitney how to use an incentive spirometer (IS). How will the nurse tell Mrs. Whitney to use the IS, and what will the nurse explain as the rationale for IS use postoperatively?

6. Mrs. Whitney is discharged from the post-anesthesia care unit (PACU) following her lumpectomy and lymph node dissection. Now that she is in your care on the nursing unit, discuss what you will assess.

7. Identify five postoperative nursing diagnoses to consider for Mrs. Whitney. List the diagnoses in order of priority.

8. In the immediate postoperative period prior to removal of the Jackson-Pratt (JP) drain, how

should the nurse assist Mrs. Whitney to position her left arm?

9. The nurse hangs a sign above Mrs. Whitney's bed to alert other members of the health care team about interventions to maintain Mrs. Whitney's safety and prevent complications of her surgery. Discuss what the sign should say.

10. The nurse gives Mrs. Whitney contact information for "Reach to Recovery." Discuss the support services available through this program.

11. Mrs. Whitney is going home today. The nurse is teaching her about possible complications of her surgery. Explain what lymphedema is, the chances of developing lymphedema, and its manifestations. Identify at least two other complications the nurse will include in the discharge teaching.

12. Discuss why tamoxifen is prescribed as part of Mrs. Whitney's treatment plan.

13. Mrs. Whitney asks about the adverse effects of tamoxifen. Create a list of the possible common and potentially life-threatening adverse effects of this medication. What instructions should you include regarding sexual activity?

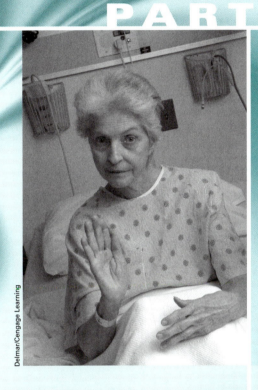

PART TWELVE

Delmar/Cengage Learning

Multi-System Failure

GENDER

Female

AGE

74

SETTING

- Intensive care unit

ETHNICITY

- White American

CULTURAL CONSIDERATIONS

PREEXISTING CONDITIONS

- Chronic obstructive pulmonary disease (COPD); hypertension; myocardial infarction (MI) 2 years ago; type 2 diabetes

COEXISTING CONDITION

COMMUNICATION

DISABILITY

SOCIOECONOMIC

- Retired veterinarian; lives at home with her husband and two dogs

SPIRITUAL/RELIGIOUS

PHARMACOLOGIC

- Claforan IV; furosemide IV; Dopamine drip

LEGAL

ETHICAL

ALTERNATIVE THERAPY

PRIORITIZATION

DELEGATION

MULTI-SYSTEM FAILURE

Level of Difficulty: Difficult

Overview: The client in this case has recently been admitted to the intensive care unit (ICU) with a diagnosis of septic shock. The causes of septic shock and its effect on body systems will be discussed. Priority nursing diagnoses will be determined.

Client Profile

Mrs. Bagent was admitted to the medical unit of the hospital 3 days ago with pneumonia and heart failure. Upon admission, the client was having difficulty breathing and had an elevated temperature and white blood cell count (WBC). Claforan IV was ordered to treat the pneumonia. Her weight had increased by 6 pounds in the 5 days preceding admission and she had significant swelling in her lower extremities. Mrs. Bagent was receiving IV furosemide (Lasix) twice a day. She became very short of breath while ambulating to the bathroom. To promote rest, an indwelling urinary catheter was inserted. During the last 24 hours her condition deteriorated and she was transferred to the intensive care unit (ICU).

Case Study

Mrs. Bagent was admitted to the ICU seven hours ago in septic shock. Her last set of vital signs were blood pressure 82/66, pulse 82, labored respirations of 32 per minute, tympanic temperature 101.2°F (38.4°C) and her oxygen saturation is 90% on 6 liters of oxygen via mask. Mrs. Bagent's skin is pale and moist, her radial pulse is rapid and thready, capillary refill is 3 seconds, and she is complaining of nausea. The nurse auscultates crackles and wheezes in all lung fields and her bowel sounds are hypoactive. Mrs. Bagent is restless and has difficulty answering questions at times because of slight confusion. The physician has ordered her urine output to be measured every hour; her last hourly output was 18 mL.

Questions

1. Define shock. Discuss the potential causes of septic shock; and state at least 3 risk factors for developing septic shock.

2. Shock affects all body systems. Discuss the signs and symptoms shock produces in the following systems: respiratory, cardiovascular, neurological, and hematological. Elaborate on the specific considerations for Mrs. Bagent in regard to each system.

3. The physician evaluating Mrs. Bagent asks the nurse what her pulse pressure is. What is a pulse pressure and why is it of concern?

4. Discuss the cellular changes that occur when a patient is in shock.

5. A Dopamine drip has been ordered.

Part A: Discuss what this medication is for, and side effects that the nurse must monitor for.

Part B: The physician orders Dopamine 8 mcg/kg/minute. Pharmacy brings the nurse a bag of Dopamine 800 mg in 500 mL of 0.9% NaCl. Mrs. Bagent's weight is 135 pounds. At what rate should the nurse program the IV pump to run (mL/hr)?

6. Mrs. Bagent's urine output is being monitored every hour. Her last hourly urine output (UO) was 18 mL. What is a goal UO? Discuss why her UO is low.

7. List five priority nursing diagnoses for Mrs. Bagent.

8. Nutritional support is very important for Mrs. Bagent. Discuss why a dietician consult is a priority and why nutritional support should occur as soon as possible.

9. Multiple Organ Dysfunction Syndrome (MODS) can occur in septic shock if perfusion to tissues cannot be restored. Discuss the signs and symptoms of MODS and treatment options.

Index

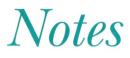

Notes

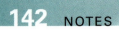